Understanding and Addressing Sexual Attraction to Children

Paedophiles exist and we must develop ways of living with this fact while ensuring that children are kept safe. This ground-breaking book demystifies the field of adult sexual attraction to children, countering the emotionality surrounding the topic of paedophilia in the popular media by careful presentation of research data and interview material. Addressing how we can work together to reduce sexual offending in this population, *Understanding and Addressing Adult Sexual Attraction to Children* bridges the gulf in understanding between those who want to protect children and those who feel sexual attraction to children – and recognises that they are sometimes the same people.

Sarah D. Goode provides an overview of the topic by defining the term 'paedophile' and discussing how many adults there may be in the general population who find themselves sexually attracted to children. She looks at how the Internet has acted as an enabler, with an explosion of child pornography and 'pro-paedophile' websites. Drawing on data from a sample of fifty-six self-defined paedophiles living in the community, she explores themes including self-identity, the place of fantasy and the forms of support available to paedophiles. Her research highlights the scale of debate within the 'online paedophile community' about issues such as the morality of sexual contact with children and encouragement to maintain a law-abiding lifestyle. Throughout, she draws careful distinctions between sexual attraction to children and sexual contact with children. The book concludes with a valuable discussion on how adult sexual contact harms children and examples of a range of initiatives which work to protect children and prevent offending.

Suitable for all professionals who work with children or sexual offenders, this book gives clear guidance on what one needs to know and do to ensure children are kept safe. It will also be of interest to students studying child protection, paedophilia and child sexual abuse within other social science disiplines.

Sarah D. Goode, a qualified occupational therapist, holds a doctorate in sociology from the University of Warwick and is Director of the Research and Policy Centre for the Study of Faith and Well-being in Communities and a Senior Lecturer in Social Care and in Community Development at the University of Winchester, UK.

Understanding and Addressing Adult Sexual Attraction to Children

A study of paedophiles in contemporary society

Sarah D. Goode

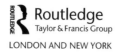

Routledge
Taylor & Francis Group

LONDON AND NEW YORK

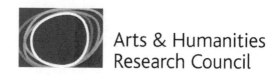

Arts & Humanities
Research Council

First published 2010
by Routledge
2 Park Square, Milton Park, Abingdon OX14 4RN

Simultaneously published in the USA and Canada
by Routledge
711 Third Avenue, New York, NY 10017

Routledge is an imprint of the Taylor & Francis Group, an informa business

© 2010 Sarah D. Goode

Typeset in Times New Roman by
Taylor & Francis Books

British Library Cataloguing in Publication Data
A catalogue record for this book is available from the British Library

Library of Congress Cataloguing in Publication Data
Goode, Sarah.
Understanding and addressing adult sexual attraction to children : a study
of paedophiles in contemporary society / Sarah Goode.
    p. cm.
1. Pedophilia. 2. Child sexual abuse. I. Title.
    HQ71.G656 2009
    362.2'7 – dc22
                2009003517

ISBN10: 0-415-44625-2 (hbk)
ISBN10: 0-415-44626-0 (pbk)
ISBN10: 0-203-87374-2 (ebk)

ISBN13: 978-0-415-44625-9 (hbk)
ISBN13: 978-0-415-44626-6 (pbk)
ISBN13: 978-0-203-87374-8 (ebk)

Contents

Tables

Preface

I am a fairly ordinary middle-aged Englishwoman, a common-or-garden-variety heterosexual, and a mother. I am also an academic involved in health and well-being. When I began the project that has resulted in this book I was angry about the fact that children continue to be sexually abused and nothing seems able to prevent this. I wanted to understand why. I was confused by the images of paedophiles presented by the media and I wanted to understand more. I hated paedophiles as much as anyone. I thought that if I ever met a paedophile I would want to kill them (even though I'm generally a pretty tolerant, pacifist Christian sort of person). But at the same time I could see that the images of deviant, cunning monsters being portrayed by the news stories and charity appeals just could not be correct. It didn't ring true. People aren't like that. So I wrote a brief exploratory paper about it for a conference. And someone got in touch with me by email and began writing to me about his thoughts and experiences. To my great surprise, I found myself communicating with a person from 'the other side of the fence', a man sexually attracted to young children. Gradually I began to correspond with other paedophiles. I arranged to meet a large group to interview them. This did not happen but instead I circulated a questionnaire and over fifty paedophiles answered it. I also met and talked to other paedophiles, only one of whom was in prison: the others were ordinary citizens getting on with their daily lives. At the same time I talked with many professionals and researchers and explored everything I could find about paedophilia, especially from a social science perspective. This book is the result.

This book is not a portrayal of how evil paedophiles are, nor is it a portrayal of how nice paedophiles are. You are invited to judge for yourself, from their own words (from published academic writing, informal online contributions, and direct quotations from research) and come to your own opinion. This book is intended to provide you with information which is not widely accessible elsewhere. The aim of my work is to draw together a huge range of material from many different disciplines to form a picture of what adult sexual attraction to children means within the context of our culture and our understandings of sexuality. This is not an easy book to read, although I have tried to make it readable. The topic of adult sexual contact with children is a painful one, and when one understands it in the context of the wider sexual and social abuses which have been perpetrated against children and women throughout the centuries, it cannot but be profoundly distressing. Indeed, it ought to be distressing. It is only by realising how badly we have gone wrong that we can begin to put things right. The conclusions are stark but I hope that they will go some way towards helping us all to create new and better ways of living safely and lovingly in this world.

If you want the message of this book in a nutshell, it is this: adult sexual contact with children should be prevented but punishing an individual for his sexual attraction rather than his actual behaviour is counterproductive; all of us adults need to behave in a much more mature and responsible way, so that all of our children can have happy childhoods, free from harm. Hating paedophiles seems easier, but doesn't keep children safe.

Acknowledgements and dedication

I would like to acknowledge the many interactions I have had with so many people in the process of completing this book and, in particular, the following individuals with all of whom I have had correspondence, whether during the process of negotiating ethics approval before conducting the research, during the course of the research and/or during the writing up of the book. All the people named below have contributed in some way or another in the lengthy work which has culminated in this book. Individuals have come from many different perspectives – from radical libertarian positions, strongly conservative positions, all points in between and many points outside such a continuum. The presence of any individual's name in the list of acknowledgements should in no way be taken as any indication of their views or of any endorsement by them of any statement expressed in this book. The views expressed in this book are my sole responsibility, except where clearly attributed.

Some of these individuals deserve salutes for courage and for courtesy and integrity in the face of great stress in their personal lives; some deserve big hugs, bunches of flowers and kisses for kindness, support and encouragement; some deserve humble acknowledgement of their inspiration and intellectual contributions. Some deserve all three! And for a book such as this, my recognition of the support given is no mere convention: academic support was a desperately real and urgent necessity in a context where I had to battle years of opposition and where at times it looked as though I would need to resign my tenure to pursue this research. I was prevented from meeting almost all the paedophile contributors face to face, in manoeuvres which were at times absurd and cowardly – an egregious example of moral panic. Sometimes, just a positive word at the right moment was all that was needed to keep me going, and I hope this book will be some small token in recognition of every act of kindness and courage. For everyone who helped with this book, and who encouraged, inspired and kept me going – thank you!

The anonymous project-management group, facilitators and contributors who made possible the Minor-Attracted Adults (MAA) online survey and associated research; the anonymous reviewers for the Arts and Humanities Research Council (AHRC) research proposal and the book proposal; Grace

McInnes, Eloise Cook, Khanam Virjee and the team at Routledge; members of B4U-ACT; DCI Mark Ashthorpe and members of Hampshire Constabulary; Alma Jones, Dr Gary Jones, Jo Brown and colleagues at the University of Winchester; Professor Sandra Drower, Dr Colin Haydon and members of the University of Winchester Faculty Ethics Committee; Professor Martin Barker; Dr Helen Betts; Professor Andrew Blake; Kevin Brown; Dr Audrey Chamberlain; 'Clayboy'; Professor Graham Crow; 'Darren'; David; Dr Francine Dolins; Douglas, Jane Fisher; 'Paul Fisher'; Professor Frank Furedi; Professor Ivor Gaber; Dr Hazel Gant; Professor Frans Gieles; Professor Lelia Green; Professor Richard Green; Dr Diederik Janssen; Professor Philip Jenkins; 'Kea', Professor James Kincaid; 'Howard Kline'; 'Daniel Lievre'; 'Mesmerised'; Claire Morris; Tom O'Carroll; Tink Palmer; Professor Nigel Parton; Professor Ken Plummer; Dr Judith Reisman; Professor Barry Richards; Dr Paul Rolph and Jenny Rolph; 'Rookiee'; Margaret Rose; Dr Gerard Schäfer; Professor Elizabeth Stuart; 'Dylan Thomas'; Dr Glenn Wilson; and Dr Richard Yuill.

In particular, I would like to thank the following individuals specifically for reading and commenting on sections of the book as it progressed: Andrew Blake, Judith Golberg, David, Judith Reisman, 'Kea', Jim Kincaid, Mark Ashthorpe, Liz Stuart, Philip Jenkins, and Barry Richards.

I would like to note that, during the course of this research, I have also had brief but helpful contact with the following individuals: Helen Drewery (Society of Friends); Kurt Eisgruber (solicitor); Xavier von Erck (Perverted Justice); Marcus Erooga, Darren Bishopp, Roger Kennington and Dr Elspeth Quayle (members of the National Organisation for the Treatment of Abusers); Gillian Finch (CISters); Donald Findlater (Lucy Faithfull Foundation); Professor David Finkelhor (CSA expert); Jane Fisher (Diocese of Winchester); Fran Henry (founder, Stop It Now!); Chris Langham (British actor); Suzie Metcalfe (Hampshire Probation Service); William Armstrong Percy III (author); James T. Sears (editor, Journal of LGBT Youth); Ray Wyre (deceased June 2008, Ray Wyre Associates); Alistair Wright (solicitor).

The completion of this project would not have been possible without the support of the Department of Health and Social Care, the Faculty of Social Sciences, the Research and Policy Centre for the Study of Faith and Well-being in Communities, and the Centre for Research and Knowledge Transfer (RKT), all based at my institution, the University of Winchester.

Statistics on sexual offending in England and Wales are from the Ministry of Justice, whom I thank for their kind assistance. The analysis and writing up of my research was enabled by a semester of research leave funded by the University of Winchester for which I express my sincere thanks.

A further semester of research leave was funded by the AHRC, for which again I would like to express sincere thanks.

This book is dedicated to Andrew, Michael and Jasmine, with an extra big hug to Judith as well, who started it all off.

1   Understanding paedophiles

Introduction

This book is unusual. It presents a view from a world which has never previously been discussed or written about in any depth, either at an academic or popular level, yet which paradoxically is almost instantly available to anyone with access to the Internet. The fundamental aim of this book is child protection, to understand and address adult sexual attraction to children in order to make the world a safer place for children, but I believe this book will also be of value and benefit in other ways as well. My intention is to assist in bridging the gulf in understanding between those who want to protect children and those who feel sexual attraction to children – and recognising that they are sometimes the same people. I take as a given the unspoken and painful truth that many men who access child pornography or who have sexual desire for or sexual contact with children are also likely, in their daily lives, to be working with or caring for children, maybe as professionals, maybe as parents. This book explores this issue and seeks to answer why and how they might be the same men – and what we can do about it. The aim of the book is to counter the emotionality surrounding the topic of paedophilia in the popular media by careful presentation of research data and interview material.

This book draws on original research with paedophiles living ordinary lives in the community and has been written as a direct response to the portrayals of paedophilia and child sexual abuse which one finds being presented every day in the media, in fund-raising charity campaigns, in educational and training materials for professionals, and in textbooks. Such portrayals often appear simplistic and psychologically naive. They ask us to believe in what amounts to almost two-dimensional cardboard cut-outs, evil monsters utterly unrelated to everyday life. And yet what we all know is that, whenever the subject is researched and whenever statistics are gathered, over and over again we find that shockingly high numbers of children aged under sixteen are sexually abused. The figure for boys is approximately 10 to 11 per cent (Cawson *et al.* 2000; Itzin 2006). For girls it is somewhere around 21 to 25 per cent (Itzin 2006; Cawson *et al.* 2000). Globally, the World Health

Organisation has found that 150 million girls and 73 million boys have experienced forced sexual intercourse and other forms of sexual violence involving physical contact before the age of eighteen (WHO 2002). Common sense tells us that if that many children are being sexually abused, then we must know the perpetrators – we must be living with them. They are not rare and horrific monsters out there lurking in the undergrowth, ready to pounce on our unwary children. They are living with us. And we must learn to understand them.

There are already many studies on the subject of adult sexual attraction to children, covering the topics of child sexual abuse, child pornography, sexology, sexual disorders and sexual deviance, children's sexuality and sexual politics, among others. However, the approach taken by this book differs significantly from previous publications with regard to its attitude towards paedophiles (adults who find themselves sexually attracted to children). There is no assumption in this book that paedophiles are pathological, deviant, criminal or evil. There is not even an assumption that they are different from us or that we have to account specifically either for their sexual attraction to children or for their choice to act on their sexual desires. Indeed, one of the aspects I am most interested in exploring is rather the choice not to act on one's sexual desires towards children – a hitherto-unexamined dynamic.

The aim throughout this book is to distinguish carefully between involuntary desires and voluntary actions and thus between being sexually attracted to children and acting on that attraction. This is a distinction often lost. Many writers working in this area seem either to dismiss entirely any attempt at empathy with those adults who are sexually attracted to children, or else, where empathy is expressed, to empathise to such a degree that it overrides any concern for children. To date, most books specifically addressing the experiences of paedophiles have been written by male authors (Rossman 1976; O'Carroll 1980; Wilson and Cox 1983; Sandfort 1987; Li *et al.* 1990; Feierman 1990; Plummer 1995; although see Yates 1978 and Levine 2002 for largely sympathetic texts written by women) and in such books it is often noticeable how very little understanding is expressed of what children – both boys and girls – need at various stages of their development: the focus of empathy tends to be exclusively on the adult male. In my work, the primary focus of my concern is children but this does not exclude the rest of us – we all were children once, and we look forward to all our children one day becoming mature and loving adults.

This book is therefore different from previous texts in this field because, it is hoped, it steers a path between the Scylla of demonising paedophiles and the Charybdis of trivialising and exonerating criminal and abusive behaviour. Paedophiles exist and we must learn to live with them in full awareness. This book aims to assist us in moving towards a realistic acceptance of that situation. Each chapter contributes to the goal of demystifying the whole field of adult sexual attraction to children, so that as a society we can all take a greater level of responsibility for protecting children from sexual abuse.

This opening chapter starts, in Section I, with an autobiographical account of David, a story of a life experience which, until now, has been entirely invisible and silent. David's story offers a way to help us begin to understand paedophilia in contemporary society. This is followed, in Section II, by a discussion on how the concept of 'paedophilia' developed and how it may be defined. This leads, in Section III, to an exploration into the vexed question of how many paedophiles there may be, and the ways in which such a question may be addressed.

Having set out basic information on what a 'paedophile' is and how many there may be, Chapter 2 then provides an opening into the hidden world of online paedophiles. It is with the rise of the Internet that social concern over paedophilia has been transformed. This chapter explores the world of the 'Darknet' where contacts can be made and files shared and downloaded under conditions of extreme secrecy, allowing the trade in child pornography to flourish. This is far from being the only or perhaps even the most significant transformation which the Internet has enabled, however. Arguably more important for many adults sexually attracted to children has been the creation of the online paedophile community. The Internet offers a resource for previously isolated paedophiles to learn about others who share their desires. More than that, it provides a way to communicate anonymously, to discuss experiences and beliefs, to build self-identities and a sense of community, and to advocate for greater understanding and tolerance. This advocacy has not been without its critics, however, and Chapter 2 ends with a brief look at anti-paedophile activism which radically changed online pro-paedophile activism, starting in 2006.

The online paedophile community introduced in Chapter 2 is the basis for the research project at the heart of this book, and Chapter 3 sets out the origins of this project. The idea for the Minor-Attracted Adults (MAA) Daily Lives Research Project first came about by chance but, having decided to research this area, it took tenacity to fight my way over many months to the point where I was finally permitted to gather the data. This chapter documents some of the factors which made this project such a struggle. It sets out in particular the ethical and methodological challenges which were posed by the subject matter and by the requirement to research volunteers through an online survey rather than through face-to-face interviewing. It is likely that when future researchers come to read this chapter in the years ahead they will scratch their heads in disbelief at the level of 'moral panic' engendered in researching paedophiles, and this chapter therefore also provides an important historical account of what it felt like to be caught up in such hysteria.

Chapter 4 provides more methodological detail on the actual conduct of the research (and copies of the research tools used in the project are reproduced in the Appendices, for future researchers who may wish to duplicate or build on this research). Since the focus of the research was not paedophiles known to the authorities (in prison or in treatment) but people living ordinary lives in the community, an essential aspect of this project was the collaboration of members of the 'online paedophile community' themselves. It was only through the support, endorsement and active cooperation of certain individuals that the research was able to be conducted at all. This was of course both a strength and a liability, and some key features of my research relationships are discussed. The aims, methodology and conduct of the research project have been set out in as transparent a manner as possible so that the findings from the project can be understood within the context of how the data were obtained. The unique nature of this research project, and the specific 'situated knowledge' which I myself bring as researcher, provide strengths and limitations which each reader may wish to evaluate individually: thus as full a description as possible has been provided of the research process.

From Chapter 5 onwards, the focus of the book is on the data provided by the MAA Daily Lives Research Project. It has not been possible to do justice to the full amount of data provided by respondents and therefore it has been decided to draw out and present in depth some of the most important topics, giving ample opportunity for direct quotation from the respondents themselves. These chapters therefore allow, as far as possible, the 'voice of the paedophile' to be heard directly, providing exact quotations from the maximum number of respondents in response to each key research question. These are also supplemented in a few cases by direct quotation from emails or interview-transcript from self-defined paedophiles, where these gave additional comments on the topic. Basic demographic data are given in Chapter 5, and then Chapter 6 turns to the question of self-identity, exploring the ways in which the online paedophile community may provide ways for individuals sexually attracted to children to construct and maintain a positive self-image. Chapter 7 addresses the topic of sexual attraction and the fantasy life of the respondents, providing a unique glimpse into their sexual and romantic desires. Chapter 8 turns to the question of support and examines whether respondents looked to any sources outside themselves for support and, if so, whether their sources of support were entirely from within the paedophile community or whether they could rely on family members, friends or people from the wider community. The question of support is strongly linked to the issue of maintaining a non-offending, law-abiding lifestyle and debates on this and other aspects of being a paedophile are discussed in Chapter 9, on the key issues and debates which appear to be most discussed in the online paedophile community.

Chapters 10 and 11 discuss the implications of these findings. First, Chapter 10 looks at the ways in which attitudes are played out in real life, with consequences which profoundly harm children. Two case studies are presented: the first identifies the ways in which those who wish to bring perpetrators to justice are marginalised, silenced and ostracised, and thus how we – as a society – fail to prevent the abuse of children. The second case study looks at the experiences of one paedophile, whom I believe to be still active in offending, and the reasons given by him for not seeking help. Thus Chapter 10 looks at the failure of child protection from the perspectives of both a concerned bystander and an actual perpetrator. But are we not all concerned bystanders? With sexual abuse affecting something in the region of one in every four girls and one in every ten or more boys (Itzin 2006), none of us can imagine that we are not involved. Chapter 11 attempts to get to grips with this reality, identifying the conclusions arising from the MAA Daily Lives Project and suggesting some ways in which we can address the challenges that are raised, so that protection and security for all children can finally begin to be a reality and not merely an ineffectual hope.

But, first, let us meet David and learn about his experiences.

Section I: David

David's story will never hit the headlines, but it is one we need to hear. It is a story of our time, and a story of profound sadness and pain. It tells us much about our dread and horror of paedophilia. It is for David and others like him, as well as for all the children, that this book has been written. This autobiographical account was given to me in response to the final question I asked in my research project. The question was 'Are there any other questions I should have asked you, or any other information you would like me to know?' David suggested that I should have asked 'Have you ever considered suicide and, if so, how close did you get?' He then went on to write about his own experiences. In the edited extract presented here, David paints a detailed and vivid picture of how it feels, as a lonely, frightened teenager, to slowly come to the horrific realisation that you yourself are 'a paedophile'.

> *I remember exactly when it started. I had just turned thirteen and was doing an important exam. I remember sitting in the school hall with about 100 other pupils and like everyone else I was nervous and looking around to see if I knew anyone for moral support. As I looked around my attention was somehow drawn to this particular guy, I didn't know him but something seemed odd about him and I couldn't quite put my finger on it. I could recognise that he was a handsome guy but there seemed to be something a small bit more interesting about him. I looked over once or twice during the exam a little puzzled but afterwards I didn't really think anymore of it but still, anytime I was asked during the summer 'How was the exam?' I thought to myself 'Wasn't it odd that I thought that guy was odd?'*
>
> *When I joined a new school, to my surprise, the guy I thought was 'odd' was there as well. As time went by and I settled into my new surroundings and got to know new people and started making new friends, I began to notice this guy more and more. It got to a point one night when I was in bed that I started thinking about him and suddenly out of nowhere I imagined kissing him! I remember it well because it sent a shiver up my spine as I thought to myself that this was certainly not right, what worried me most was not so much the fact I imagined kissing a guy but the fact that it seemed to feel nice. The fright of it put it out of my mind and I vowed*

never to think of it again. Besides, I like women, they're sexy and imagining being with Pamela Anderson felt nice too.

But now, not only was this guy in my school and my classroom, he was also in my social group of friends. I soon enough started to figure that I had an attraction to this guy because I was starting to have sexual fantasies about him. They felt really nice but I knew there was something going very wrong. I made sure that I never looked at an attractive guy, I learnt very quickly to always casually look the other direction to the point where it became almost second nature to me. After a time, I could see by the way classmates and friends interacted with me that it seemed no one could see it in me at all and I started to relax a little. 'I'm not gay, I'm just straight and confused' I thought. 'It's just hormones and all I have to do is wait until they calm down, I knew I wasn't gay!' That held me up for the rest of the year.

As I turned fourteen I was still in the group of friends with the guy I was attracted to. His presence was an uncomfortable reminder of what was wrong inside of me. As time went by the 'hormone theory' defence was starting to wear thin and I started to consider that perhaps maybe this is it, maybe I am actually gay. For the vast majority of my time I just basically ignored it and just got on with life. By the time my fifteenth year came around 'hormone theory' was hanging by a thread and I guess the shock of having homosexuality in the first place had started to wear thin. I reckoned if those hormones were going to ever settle down they would have settled by now surely. I started to slowly accept that I had homosexuality in me, I guess it's not the worst thing in the world. I was still attracted to women but it only seemed about 75/25. At some point I decided to end the remaining conflict and worry inside me. Basically it went along the lines of a compromise, I said to myself, 'Right, I accept that I am seemingly stuck with homosexuality, so here's the deal. Homosexuality, you can go over to that corner and fantasise about whatever you want and I'll go over to this corner and live my life through heterosexuality the way I want and we'll just pretend we never met, full stop.' I still felt a little cheated but there didn't seem like there was any other way of dealing with it. Life went on as normal and as time went on it just didn't seem to matter as much as it used to, I became used to it and as such it was easily ignored.

I felt happy enough as I turned sixteen. But something had changed. As much as I was peacefully ignoring homosexuality, I couldn't help but make a number of strange observations. Observation number one was: Why is it that the couple of guys in my classes that I always thought seemed attractive, are now definitely not as attractive as they used be? It seemed very odd. Observation number two was: If I'm gay then why is it that I'm not attracted to Brad Pitt? I can see he's a very handsome guy and I've heard he's a gay idol but now that I take a look I find that I have no attraction for him or in fact any adult male no matter how good-looking. Observation number 3: Disturbingly, why is it that the only guys who do seem attractive are the ones aged around twelve or thirteen? In fact, they seem more like boys than anything else. I started to get a very bad feeling that something was going very, very wrong. The more I looked at it the more worried I was getting. I simply didn't know what or why this was happening to me.

That was the year when Father Smith hit the front page of every newspaper my parents brought home with them. A new evil was born from an inferno of horror and fear and its name was Paedophilia. I had never heard that word before that. Father Smith was a paedophile and as the newspaper explained, a paedophile was a person who had an attraction to children. Father Smith had sex with young boys. The only people I seemed to be attracted to were boys. At first a wave of utter disbelief and confusion passed over me. There is no way on God's green earth I would do anything like the horror Father Smith perpetrated on those boys. I started to think that whatever Father Smith had it must be different from what I have. I mean, why did he do those things? Why would you hurt any boy? It simply didn't make any sense whatsoever. As the weeks and months passed by I read every article about paedophilia from the papers my parents brought home. I made sure I was very careful not to let my parents or anyone else in my family see me read these articles. One Sunday, in an in-depth investigation of paedophilia, the newspaper finally explained why people like Father Smith were so cruel to children. Paedophilia is an 'incurable psychological disease' it wrote, and it is only a matter of time, circumstance and opportunity before a paedophile strikes his victim.

As the realisation of what this meant set in, it started to dawn on me that paedophilia, as a disease, must be like a cancer. A cancer of the mind. What I knew about cancer was that it's a disease that starts off very small. So small you wouldn't even know it was there. As time goes by it begins to consume everything around it to the point that by the time you find out you have it, it would be, more or less, too late to do anything about it. Then it would kill you. I realised that paedophilia had started off small. I didn't even realise I had it all this time. I thought it was homosexuality. I'm only sixteen now and that's why I'm still a good person but as time goes by paedophilia would slowly consume all that was good and decent inside me, then it would only be a matter of circumstance and opportunity before I start raping, beating and destroying boys too! I would become as evil as Father Smith. There will be nothing I could do to stop it. Every night these thoughts would circle my head time and time again. Fear started to grow slowly at first but very surely. 'Something's coming' I thought. Some kind of remorseless and shameless joy from raping and beating innocent boys.

Night after night alone in my bedroom fear was growing and growing, I could feel it. There was such a hatred for paedophiles being expressed by every newspaper and the thing about it was, they were right to feel that way about Father Smith and people like him. People like me. I suddenly realised at this point, that everyone in this life, my friends, my family, my mum and dad, all hate me too, it's just that they don't know it yet! I started to feel isolated from everyone around me. To feel alone in this world, to face a battle with a cancer I might never win.

To walk around with a worried face or to act any differently would draw questions from parents, teachers or friends. Questions I most certainly had no answers to and a personal issue I could afford no one in my life to find out about. When I was around people I literally reverted back to my normal everyday self. What I thought was homosexuality had already trained me to do this. I felt and displayed no fear or concern to anyone and dealt with everyone and everything the way I would as if this thing didn't exist.

At night-time, however, when I was alone in my room, that's when Pandora's box would open and all hell rode out from it. How anyone could live with the shame of sexually abusing boys is one question. But how could anyone continue to live with the shame of knowing they are destined to destroy boys is quite another. I asked myself, 'Is it right for me to continue to live knowing what I'll end up doing to boys in the future?' I felt the answer but didn't say it. Suicide had entered the equation. Suicide brought with it the absolute, guaranteed and undisputable fact that I would never in this life harm even one boy ever, full stop.

I knew that if I didn't find my way out of paedophilia and soon then I was going to die by my own hand. The search was on. I don't remember anyone around me ever talking about it even though I tried to listen for it. I went back into the newspapers reading and rereading the articles, trying to 'read between the lines'. I didn't know exactly what I was looking for but I thought I'd know if I found it. But as time went by there was a gathering sense that I wouldn't find anything in the newspapers. I had read these papers for over two years now and the stories were always the same, time and again. I was slowly losing hope that I'd find something to save me. Suicide was with me night after night. As the weeks went by fear was ebbing away to the sorrow of slowly accepting my fate. I had done everything I could, I've done the best I can, I've explored all the options. There just wasn't any way out.

I started to think more about the concept of suicide and what it meant. It meant I was never going to hurt any boy, guaranteed. I then began to realise that what I was going to do through suicide was to actually save boys and anyone who actively does something to save another, especially children, is called 'a hero'. The term 'a paedophile' means 'a destroyer of children'. But I'm going to be saving boys not hurting them. It means I'm not 'a paedophile' in any way, shape or form. While it's clear beyond doubt that no one in this life could ever love 'a paedophile' it is, however, just as clear that everyone in this life certainly loves 'a hero'. Everyone loves a hero! Everyone loves ... me! Of course they do! Everything was perfect. Everything was beautiful. Everything made brilliant sense, all questions answered. Suicide isn't a decision, it's an understanding. A perfect understanding. The next day I when I left my room I was walking around on a cloud. I could barely keep the smile off my face. Everything felt so different, so bright. The horrific disease had gone so I could find no fault within myself and therefore no fault in anyone else either. Everything was perfect. After a couple of days of walking around feeling great I knew the time had come to plan how I was going to commit suicide. In my room that night I settled down to the task of finding a way to commit suicide.

There seemed to be many ways to do it from drug overdose to walking in front of a bus. I quickly enough generated a small list of priorities that a suicide method must fulfil. Priority number one: it must at all costs be guaranteed. Priority number two: it has to be quick. Priority number three: if possible it has to be painless. The best way seems to be slitting my wrists with a razor in the bathroom. This seems perfect. It's absolutely guaranteed beyond doubt, it will take five minutes maximum, it's quick and of course the deeper the cut the less the pain. Now that I picked the method and the place it was now time to set the date. I chose a date about a month and a half away. All I had to do now was sit and wait. I sat there on the eve of the appointed day with the razor in my hand but I just couldn't do it!

While it most certainly wasn't the last time I came close to suicide in those first few years, no other time had such an impact on me. My psychology had collapsed and I emotionally and logically flat-lined with no more ability to function than to just show people what they wanted to see so I could get to the end of my day and disappear under the pillow. The story from that suicide attempt to now is one I would call a slow rebuild of personal ideology and understanding of how my life works.

David's experiences as a suicidal teenager serve as a powerful reminder of why this book needs to be written and why, as professionals and lay people, we need to know the information that this book provides.

My goal in writing this book is to make available the information that will help us, as members of society, to understand what it is like to be sexually attracted to children. The information in this book should help those, like David, who find themselves experiencing a sexual attraction they did not choose and who are worried that, in consequence, they may turn into the 'evil monsters' portrayed in the media. This book is also for all those who are involved in this issue in some way, whether as professionals, lay helpers or friends, who work with or care about people who are sexually attracted to children. It is also for those who may have known a paedophile themselves when they were a child, or who experienced sexual contact with an adult, and who want to understand their own experiences in more depth. Finally, this book is for all those children, past, present and future, whose lives are harmed by the sexual behaviour of others. It is my sincere hope that this book will go some way towards keeping them safer, and building a more protective society in which we can all take responsibility for our own actions.

Section II: Definitions of paedophilia

As we can see from David's account, information which could help someone understand sexual attraction to children can be extremely hard to find, with desperate consequences. The remainder of this chapter sets out some basic facts to help us understand more about paedophilia. The following section provides information on the medical and historical understandings of this condition and some of the pragmatic and political difficulties inherent in defining it. The final section gives an overview of what we know about how many paedophiles there may be.

There is a clear distinction to be made at the outset between child sexual abuse (adult sexual contact with children below the legal age of consent) and paedophilia (adult sexual attraction to children below the legal age of consent). Child sexual abuse, under a variety of terms, has existed for as long as there have been legal definitions of the age of consent. Prior to that, and in any situations where legal ages of consent do not exist, children will still be vulnerable to sexual abuse and rape but the recognition that harm is occurring may be lacking. Paedophilia is, strictly speaking, in a separate conceptual category to child sexual abuse. It is defined as a medical condition similar to other psychosexual disorders or 'paraphilias' (disorders of sexual function). The contemporary definition of paedophilia, therefore, is tied up with its medical diagnosis and clinical treatment. Paedophilia, as we currently understand it, is the medical diagnosis of a fixed sexual orientation which may or may not manifest itself in actual behaviour towards a child. The technical diagnostic term 'paedophilia erotica' was first put forward by a German medical doctor, Krafft-Ebing, in the nineteenth century. A gifted and influential scientist, Baron Richard von Krafft-Ebing was appointed Professor of Psychiatry at Strasbourg at the early age of thirty-two and contributed to his field by taking on the task of carefully describing, analysing and classifying the varieties of mental illness he observed. He was fascinated by sex and all its multifarious variations. He analysed the cases of unusual sexuality that he came across as examples of 'degeneration', in other words as being due to a pre-existing biological base, an impaired genetic inheritance, rather than to individual moral choice, although he did also recognise a distinction between those who were 'degenerate' or fixed in their sexual desires and those who chose to experiment. He discussed these variations in the form of a series of case studies and published his findings in his major work, *Psychopathia Sexualis*. This book was first published in 1886 and went through many editions, reprints and translations, with the most recent reissue of the English edition being in 1998. The impact of this book has been immense: it is from the *Psychopathia Sexualis* that we have the terms sadism, masochism, fetishism, necrophilia, homosexuality, heterosexuality and paedophilia. As well as introducing a whole host of new classifications to sexual experience, Krafft-Ebing made a further significant contribution to medicine, to forensic psychiatry and to the legal system, by asserting that sexual deviation was a medical rather than a judicial problem. For example, he argued that homosexuals were not criminal so much as diseased: therefore they were in need of treatment rather than punishment. From the work of Krafft-Ebing and others, over the course of the late nineteenth and into the twentieth century, emerged the new field of sexology.

While many other nineteenth-century medical and scientific classifications and concepts have fallen into disuse and been replaced by more developed theories, it is notable (and rather curious) that these early sexological terms, far from disappearing, have become increasingly well known and recognised. Over 100 years later, Krafft-Ebing's technical classification of one obscure sexual anomaly, paedophilia, has become one of the most well-worn of the stock-in-trade labels used by tabloid journalism.

Paedophilia is often linked, both by its opponents and its proponents, to another of Krafft-Ebing's diagnoses, homosexuality and, for proponents of paedophilia at least, there would seem to be clear benefits to this linkage. Homosexuality is a sexual classification which has moved from the realm of the criminal (and thus punished) to the realm of the sick (and thus treated) and then, more recently, into the realm of the normal everyday lifestyle choice. Proponents of paedophilia as a lifestyle choice therefore look to the recent history of the decriminalisation of male homosexuality (female homosexuality has typically never been criminalised to the same extent) as a harbinger of the route that the diagnosis of paedophilia may take. A brief review of the history of the 'diagnosis' of homosexuality therefore serves as a way into understanding some of debates on the diagnosis and definitions of paedophilia. While homosexual behaviour is still illegal in some forty countries around the world (Nuffield 2008), within most countries it has now been accepted as neither illegal nor a mental disorder.

Throughout the world, most countries rely on one of two major classification systems for diagnoses of mental disorders: either the World Health Organisation's *International Classification of Diseases, Mental Disorders Section* (the *ICD*, currently the tenth edition 1994) or the American Psychiatric Association's *Diagnostic and Statistical Manual for Mental Disorders* (the *DSM*, currently the fourth revised edition 2000). These two key texts essentially define which mental disorders actually exist and which do not and, as a corollary, which can therefore be paid for and treated under health insurance. Whether a condition is listed as a 'disorder' or not has the power to fundamentally alter an individual's life (are they 'sick' or not? Do they need 'treatment'?). It can also fundamentally alter the culture surrounding that individual (are they accepted as 'normal' or rejected as 'sick' by those around them?). It is not surprising therefore that the classification of homosexuality as a mental disorder was challenged so strongly in the 1970s. After all, there is little sense in having 'Gay Pride' if homosexuality is in fact an illness. The emergent gay rights movement in the USA used the *DSM* as a focus for political activism, and campaigners on both sides argued fiercely and acrimoniously (Bayer 1981; Bayer and Spitzer 1982) over the status of homosexuality and whether it should be retained or removed as a diagnosis. After much argument it was removed as a diagnosis in 1973 and then replaced in 1980 with the diagnosis of 'ego dystonic homosexuality' (in other words, homosexuality which causes distress to the individual). This diagnosis was then removed as well, in 1986. In 1993 it was also removed as a diagnosis from the other major system of classification, the *ICD*.

Some campaigners are keen to see a similar trajectory followed by the diagnosis of other 'paraphilias' (sexual disorders), including paedophilia. O'Donohue *et al.* (2000) review the difficulties with the diagnosis of paedophilia, while Moser and Kleinplatz (2003) go further, arguing that 'the situation of the paraphilias at present parallels that of homosexuality in the early 1970s. Without the support or political astuteness of those who fought for the removal of homosexuality, the paraphilias continue to be listed in the *DSM*'. They presented their view in a paper at a symposium hosted by the American Psychiatric Association (APA), at which, paralleling the debates in the 1970s over homosexuality, there were heated discussions over whether to remove paedophilia and other paraphilias as diagnostic categories. The APA felt so beleaguered by this onslaught they were compelled to issue a statement reasserting their position that an adult 'who engages in sexual activity with a child is performing a criminal and immoral act and this is never considered normal or socially acceptable behavior' (Oseran 2003).

One campaigner, Richard Green, a lawyer as well as a professor at both Imperial College and Cambridge University, is of note here because he was one of the original activists arguing for the removal of the diagnosis of homosexuality back in the 1970s (Green 1972). Thirty years later, he is now putting the case for the removal of the diagnosis of paedophilia (Green 2002: 469) arguing that the 'evolution of pedophilia in the different editions of *DSM* is a trip through Alice's Wonderland'. Green's paper was only one of a number of comments on whether paedophilia is a mental disorder – an entire edition of the journal *Archives of Sexual Behavior* (the official journal of the International Academy of Sex Research) was given over to the discussion, with twenty-four participants involved, but coming to no clear consensus (Gieles 2002). It is indeed the case that, since the *DSM* was first published in 1952, there have been five different attempts at developing diagnostic criteria for paedophilia, and arguably none are fully satisfactory.

The most recent version (*DSM-IV-TR,* APA 2000) has three conditions which need to be met in order for a diagnosis of paedophilia to be made. First, it requires that, over a period of at least six months, the individual has experienced recurrent, intense sexually arousing fantasies, sexual urges, or behaviours involving sexual activity with a prepubescent child or children. (The *DSM* classifies 'prepubescent' as generally meaning aged thirteen years or younger.) Second, the individual must either have acted on these sexual urges, or the sexual urges or fantasies must have caused the individual marked distress or interpersonal difficulty. Third, the individual must be aged at least sixteen years, and must be at least five years older than the child or children in the fantasies or activities. The sexual attraction may be limited only to incestuous relationships within the individual's own family. To be diagnosed, the individual need not be exclusively attracted to children. However, the *DSM* specifically excludes an individual in late adolescence who is involved in an ongoing sexual relationship with a child aged twelve or thirteen years old, although it is not clear why this exclusion is made.

As Green and others have pointed out, this diagnosis of paedophilia means that an individual may have recurrent, intense sexually arousing fantasies and sexual urges involving a prepubescent child or children but, if they do not act on them and if they do not cause marked distress or interpersonal difficulty, then that individual would not be diagnosed as having paedophilia. This does seem rather anomalous and, in fact, is not the definition of paedophilia being followed in this book, which uses a working definition of paedophilia as meaning an individual who is predominantly or exclusively sexually attracted to children below the legal age of consent, whether or not they act on that sexual attraction (and whether or not they are distressed by their attraction or have had interpersonal difficulties because of it).

Difficulties in this area seem to have no ending. In the previous version of the *DSM* (*DSM-III-R*), the criteria for the paraphilias had included a clinical significance criterion which was that 'the person has acted on these urges, or is markedly distressed by them', in recognition of the fact that the mere presence of certain sexual urges or fantasies do not necessarily warrant a diagnosis of a behaviour in an individual. In the more recent edition (*DSM-IV-TR* 2000), the wording of this criterion was adjusted so that paedophilia was now defined as comprising fantasies, sexual urges, or behaviours causing clinically significant distress or impairment in social, occupational, or other important areas of functioning. This rewording led to unexpected difficulties which the APA was then forced to address. On 18 January 2008, the APA posted on its website a clarification explaining their 'Adjustment of wording of the clinical significance criterion for the Paraphilias' (APA 2008). Here they explained that their removal of the reference to acting on urges 'was misconstrued to represent a fundamental change in the definition' of paedophilia, by seeming to exclude both those individuals who were not distressed by their urges and even those who did act on their paedophilic urges. Oops! The original wording was quickly reinstated.

What all these complex and convoluted rewordings demonstrate abundantly is the difficulty of defining paedophilia precisely. As if the definition of 'paedophilia' was not complex enough, this condition has also recently been broken down further, into the related categories of nepiophilia (also termed infantophilia) and ephebophilia (also termed hebephilia). These terms have been used for sexual attraction to babies and toddlers and sexual attraction to minors around the age of consent, respectively. For example, the term 'ephebophilia' is used by the well-known sexologist Dr John Money in his Foreword to Theo Sandfort's 1987 book *Boys on their Contacts with Men,* and Money also describes infantophilia and nepiophilia in Jay Feierman's edited compilation on *Pedophilia: Biosocial Dimensions* (1990: 451), where he says, 'If the eligible partner is an infant, "infantophilia" is the diagnostic term. If it is essential that the infant be wearing diapers, however, the Greek-derived term for the diapered infant, "nepiophilia" applies.' (We will pass over the implications of Money's use of the term 'eligible partner' to describe a baby.) It is not clear whether Money himself coined these terms, although nepiophilia (with or without the connotation of diapers) does seems to be used within the paedophile community. However, these terms do not appear to be listed in the *DSM* or *ICD,* and most online references to the terms are circular, bringing the reader back to a disputed Wikipedia article on 'Infantophilia' (Wikipedia 2008). This article was flagged, as from January 2008, as needing to be expanded, linked and verified by the use of citations; in other words, as being insufficiently scientific to comply with Wikipedia's standards as an online encyclopedia. Thus it is possible, interestingly, that these terms have been adopted, not from the medical establishment (other than possibly the work of John Money), but primarily from the paedophile community itself, where they are sometimes taken as a self-definition (for an example of this, see 'Ian' in Chapter 10).

Section III: How many paedophiles are there?

While I think I have a good grasp on my own experience and how it shaped me as the person I am now, I am aware there's lots more complexity out there in the wider issue. What's quite crippling is the lack of facts, figures and proper statistics to be able to form a proper picture of the reality out there. Picking up the odd fact or figure from newspapers or television really isn't good enough I think. However I do try to work with what I can get nevertheless. It's a problem for everyone I guess.

(David)

David is not alone in his difficulty in trying to find 'facts, figures and proper statistics' to understand adult sexual attraction to children. Having grappled with some of the practical and political difficulties inherent in trying to define paedophilia, let's look at numbers. This section now engages with the question of how many paedophiles there may be in the general population.

There are some things which are relatively easy to find out, such as the number of people at any one time who are convicted for sexual offences against children. Taking the situation in England and Wales as an example – two countries with a combined total population of 53 million people – it is interesting to see how low the figures for sexual offences actually are. The Ministry of Justice has published a set of criminal statistics covering the decade 1997 to 2006 inclusive, and most of the data on sexual offences against children are available in Table 3.13 on page 70 of the Ministry's Report (Ministry of Justice 2007). I have supplemented this published data with additional material provided directly from the Ministry (personal communication, May 2008).

To make sense of the figures, we need to separate convictions (where a person is arrested, taken to court, found guilty and sentenced) from cautions (where a person is not arrested but is given a formal caution by a police officer which is then recorded and kept on file). Also, we need to be aware of changing legislation, which affects the definition of a criminal offence and thus affects what offences are recorded and get into the statistics. The offences are usually categorised according to whether the child is female or male and whether the child is aged between birth and twelve years, thirteen and fifteen (or, for some offences, thirteen and seventeen) or eighteen years or older. The offences are usually further categorised according to whether the offender was aged under or over eighteen years at the time of the offence: this addresses the concerns that people may have that sex between a sixteen-year-old girl and her seventeen-year-old boyfriend, for example, might be inflating the sex-offender figures.

In this discussion, I will concentrate only on those offences committed against a child aged between birth and twelve years, by an offender aged over eighteen years, which involved direct sexual contact: that is, penetration, rape, attempted rape, sexual assault, unlawful sexual intercourse, incest and sexual activity where the offender is in a position of trust in relation to the child. (Offences of causing or inciting a child to engage in sexual activity have been omitted from this discussion, as has 'gross indecency' which does not specify the age of the child.) In total, there are seventeen relevant offences which could be committed against a child specified as being under thirteen years old, of which all except two (incest with a girl under thirteen, and unlawful sex with a girl under thirteen) have only applied since 2003, and thus only have figures from 2004. Since these seventeen offences came into force, there have been a total of 133, 397 and 552 convictions of adults aged over eighteen years old, during the years 2004, 2005 and 2006 respectively. These were convictions for offences including sexual activity when the adult is in a position of trust (one conviction for abuse of a boy; two convictions for abuse of a girl); attempted rape of a boy (three convictions) and attempted rape of a girl (seven convictions); penetration of a boy (eleven convictions); and incest with a female child (a total of 103 convictions between 1997 and 2006). If we add up all the convictions for direct sexual offences with a child aged less than thirteen years, from 1997 to 2006, we arrive at a grand total of 1,522 convictions over the whole decade.

Taking just the figure for 2006 (when more adults were convicted of sexual offences against children under thirteen than in any previous year of the decade), this still gives us, as we have seen, a figure of 552 convictions. If, instead of looking only at offences against children aged below thirteen years, we look at the total number of all convictions for all sexual offences against children (including against those aged sixteen and up to seventeen years in certain circumstances), this gives a figure of 2,304 for the year 2006. If we also add in the total number of cautions given for all these sexual offences (which totals 755 cautions), this gives us a grand total of 3,059 offenders who came to the attention of the police for sexual offences against children and were given either a police caution or were found guilty in a court of law.

So, out of a population of 53 million people, around 3,000 people might be cautioned or convicted of these offences annually. Since children under sixteen comprise 20.2 per cent of the population of England and Wales (Census 2001), this means that, in approximate terms, the adult population is around 40 million and therefore that, out of this adult population, approximately one out of every 13,000 adults is convicted or cautioned each year for sexual abuse of children aged up to sixteen years, of which one-sixth of these, approximately one out of every 78,000 adults, is convicted of a sexual offence against a child under thirteen. However, if we accept that sexual abuse of children is typically carried out by men rather than women (Itzin 2000), this gives an approximate prevalence of one man in every 40,000 men (thus 0.0025 per cent).

If we turn to the use of child pornography, this has been of increasing concern over the past few years, as shown for example by the international police operation known as Operation Ore which resulted in 7,000 arrests in Britain in 2003. What impact did this have on the level of cautions and convictions? In 2003, when Operation Ore was at its height, the figures from England and Wales more than doubled. From 531 in 2002, the total peaked in 2003 at 1,287 people found guilty of taking, making or possessing an indecent photograph of a child. Since 2003, the figures have settled at around 1,000 people a year: 1,162 in 2004, 1,154 in 2005 and 934 in 2006 (data from Ministry of Justice, personal communication, May 2008). So, judging by the number of individuals found guilty of child pornography offences, it would seem, as with direct sexual contact offences, to be a very small-scale phenomenon indeed.

However, this contrasts with evidence online. In the following chapter we will look at material on the Internet, including the presence of online messages offering and discussing popular 'series' of child pornography images (Jenkins 2001), 'pro-paedophile' websites and the presence of fantasy-material dealing with 'child erotica' such as erotic stories, 'doll albums', and lolicon or shotacon manga (highly sexualised cartoon portrayals of, respectively, small girls and small boys). All these phenomena indicate that there is a fairly extensive market for discussion, images, stories and other items dealing with adult sexual attraction to children. While not providing any clear answers, these forms of indicative evidence suggest intriguing questions about prevalence and about the complex interrelationship between fantasy and action.

What other forms of evidence can we draw on to answer the question 'How many paedophiles are there?' Statistical evidence is hard to come by. 'I write "1, 5, 21, 50" on the board and ask my students, 'Which is the percentage of pedophiles in the country?'.... the answer is all of them' according to psychologist Paul Okami (quoted in Levine 2002: 25). Okami believes that the proportion of (male) Americans whose primary erotic focus is prepubescent children is around 1 per cent, a figure which is broadly consonant with clinical and community studies discussed later in this section but startlingly different from the 0.0025 per cent convicted of offences.

Another form of evidence is to use data on brain structure and neuroendocrinology. This has some fascinating implications both for understanding how many paedophiles there may be in a population and also what the biochemical basis of paedophilia (or at least some aspects of it) might be. Studies have looked at how the male human brain is 'masculinised' and 'defeminised' by hormones circulating in the mother's body while the baby is still in the womb. At the embryo stage, all babies are 'female' in that, unless acted upon by specific hormones, babies develop the internal reproductive organs, external genitalia and forms of brain structure which are 'feminine' or 'female-typical'. Only in the relative presence of certain hormones and the relative absence of others will embryos develop into males. In order to become male, therefore, an embryo needs both to be actively 'masculinised' and also actively 'defeminised'.

The process of masculinisation occurs first, then defeminisation. According to biologists studying animal models (Feierman 1990; Hutchison and Hutchison 1990), the neurochemical process of masculinisation links sexuality with 'social dominance' behaviours, that is, competitive aggressiveness, active 'courtship' and 'mounting' or 'insertion' behaviours. This linking of sexuality with social dominance makes males sexually attracted to 'small', 'weak', 'young' and 'helpless' individuals (Feierman 1990: 46). Feierman suggests that the brains of paedophiles are 'extremely masculinised' (1990: 46; later Feierman adjusts this to 'slightly more masculinised than occurs in adult heterosexual males', 1990: 53), making them more likely to find extremely submissive (that is, very small, weak, young and helpless) individuals the most sexually attractive. The neurochemical process of defeminisation removes the 'female-typical' behaviour patterns (such as mammals sticking out their bottoms to encourage males to mate with them – think Marilyn Monroe, if you will) and at the same time increases the likelihood that males will find such 'feminised' behaviour sexually alluring (think of the typical heterosexual male response to Monroe). Feierman claims that paedophiles are 'slightly less defeminised' than heterosexual men (1990: 53), thus they would be less likely to be aroused by typical 'feminine' behaviours. Sociobiological explanations for human behaviour do have a rather conservative tendency to look at what *is,* and then search for explanations in unlikely places (mice, reptiles, birds and so forth) to explain and justify the social status quo; however, the two-dimensional model of embryonic brain masculinisation and brain defeminisation can both suggest why some men might find children sexually attractive and also predict, given a normal distribution curve for this biochemical process, what order of magnitude we might expect for paedophiles in a population. Feierman (1990: 51), looking only at men, suggests that 'the central tendency in evolution is to produce heterosexual males by producing an optimal amount of masculinisation and defeminisation of the male brain in utero.' When the levels of masculinisation and defeminisation are slightly skewed, homosexuality, paedophilia (to either males or females) or transsexualism will result. From this model, Feierman predicts that, in any given population of men, paedophiles will be more common than homosexuals who will in turn be more common than transsexuals. He also predicts that:

> If the distribution of the points in the model reflects differing degrees of masculinisation and defeminisation of the male brain, then there is every reason to believe that the distributions would actually be continuous across all males rather than being discontinuous around arbitrary and nonmutually exclusive categories such as 'heterosexual' and 'androphilic ephebophile' [a man attracted to adolescent boys].
>
> (Feirerman 1990: 52)

Feierman later describes this rather technically but memorably in the following way:

> [Paedophiles] are the 'by-products' of the inevitable biological variation around a selected central tendency. So that most males will 'love' children and adolescents just the right amount...some males will unfortunately love them too little and some too much. Such males, who love children and adolescents to a degree more than average or less than average, will be carried along in a population in the tails of frequency distributions. ...It is most likely, therefore, that pedo- and ephebophilia are individual, facultative proclivities that are bent out of the tails of hormonal frequency distributions around the optimum brain masculinisation and brain feminisation of the 'average male'.
>
> (Feierman 1990: 559, 563)

In other words, Feierman seems to be implicitly proposing four important hypotheses in this model:

1. Paedophilia is caused by brain chemistry arising before birth: that is, paedophiles are born, not made.
2. Paedophiles fall within a normal distribution curve for human males.
3. Paedophiles are more common than homosexuals.
4. Sexual attraction to individuals smaller and more 'feminine' than oneself (including boys and young adolescents) is part of a continuum occurring in *all* males, not just paedophiles, and thus there is no clear cut-off point between a 'paedophile' and a 'non-paedophile'.

Feierman is also, of course, conflating 'love' with sexual attraction, but, leaving that on one side, these are still some pretty hefty claims and would clearly need a great deal of substantiating evidence. Hutchison and Hutchison, for example, working for the British Medical Research Council Neuroendocrine Development and Behaviour Group and writing on 'Sexual development at the neurohormonal level: the role of androgens', are more cautious, commenting that most work so far has been carried out on animal models such as rodents and birds, as well as in-vitro experiments and that postnatal social experience 'appears to be more influential in human development than it is in the development of nonhuman species' (1990: 538). Feierman would also need to explain why, if this is an evolutionary biological process, we do not find paedophile behaviour in animals, including in primates (for evidence that we do not, see chapters in Feierman's own edited volume, 1990).

Following on from Feierman's implication that sexual attraction to children may represent a continuum within human male sexuality, a further way to approach the question of the prevalence of paedophilia is to look at what 'normal' adults – who are not defined in any way as 'paedophile' – may reveal about their sexual attraction to children. There are eight studies in total which have been conducted to date, which begin to help us answer the question of how many paedophiles there are, by looking at the responses of 'normal' men in the general adult male population (and one of the studies also included women in their study). The studies relied on three basic methods: direct self-report (what the research subjects themselves said about their sexual arousal to children); more general questionnaire responses (which included measurements such as 'sexual impulsivity' and self-esteem); and physical responses. In this research, 'physical responses' meant fitting a 'strain gauge' to the man's penis and using a machine called a 'penile plethysmograph' to measure how much his penis reacted, for example when images were shown or tapes narrating a sexual story were played. The results (especially when we compare them with the conviction/caution rate for child sexual offences) are pretty unexpected.

If we take the clinical studies first, there have been five studies in this area (discussed in Green 2002). The earliest (Freund and Costell 1970) studied forty-eight young Czech soldiers who were shown slides of young children, adolescents and adults, both male and female. All the soldiers showed penile response to adult women, forty of them (83 per cent) showed penile response to adolescent girls, and twenty-eight of the soldiers (58 per cent) showed penile response to the slides of little girls aged four to ten years old. Next, in a study five years later (Quinsey *et al.* 1975), 'normal' men's erections to pictures of pubescent and younger girls averaged 70 and 50 per cent, respectively, of their responses to adult women. Freund and Watson (1991), studying community male volunteers in a plethysmography classification study, found that 19 per cent were 'misclassified' as having an erotic preference for minors. In a control group of sixty-six males recruited from hospital staff and the community, 17 per cent showed a penile response that was pedophilic (Fedora *et al.* 1992). Finally, in the most recent study of this kind (Nagayama Hall *et al.* 1995), a sample of eighty volunteers was recruited from the general population. To explore their responses, the researchers showed the volunteers images and also used audiotapes with sexual narratives. The images and tapes referred to adult women and to girls under the age of twelve years. Sexual arousal was measured using self-report and physical measurements of penile arousal. In this presumably 'normal' community sample 20 per cent self-reported paedophilic interest and 26.25 per cent exhibited a penile response to paedophilic stimuli that equalled or exceeded their arousal to adult stimuli.

The clinical studies therefore indicate that somewhere between 17 and 58 per cent of a 'normal' sample of men (who do not describe themselves as 'paedophile') seem to be capable of being sexually aroused by young children, under the age of twelve years old. In other words, roughly one in six to more than one in every two adult men may be capable of being sexually attracted to children.

Besides these laboratory studies there have also, to date, been three surveys which used questionnaires to explore adult sexual arousal to children. The first of these (Briere and Runtz 1989) looked at a sample of nearly 200 university males, in which 21 per cent reported some sexual attraction to small children, 9 per cent described sexual fantasies involving children, 5 per cent admitted to having masturbated to sexual fantasies of children, and 7 per cent indicated they might have sex with a child if not caught. This study was followed up a few years later (Smiljanich and Briere 1996), with a questionnaire study on 279 undergraduates which included ninety-nine men and 188 women. This found 22 per cent of the male sample (and 3 per cent of the female sample) admitted 'some attraction to little children', with 14 per cent of the men using child pornography, 4 per cent masturbating to sexual fantasies involving children and 3 per cent admitting to the 'possibility of sex with child if undetected' (figures for the female sample were respectively 4 per cent, 0 per cent and 0 per cent). Both these studies made the point that any self-report of socially unacceptable phenomena is likely to underestimate it, so these figures may be conservative. The most recent study in this area used similar questions to the two previous surveys (Becker-Blease *et al.* 2006) in a self-completion questionnaire study of 531 undergraduate men. This study found only 7 per cent admitted sexual attraction to 'little children', but 18 per cent had sexual fantasies of children, with 8 per cent masturbating to those fantasies, and 4 per cent admitting that they would have sex with a child 'if no one found out'.

These questionnaire studies therefore support the laboratory findings and again suggest that somewhere in the region of one in every five men is likely to have some degree of sexual attraction to children. Remember, these survey rates were found by relying *only* on what the volunteers decided to disclose to the researchers. It's probable that, even when anonymity and confidentiality are absolutely guaranteed, a proportion of people who are asked questions such as this on a written questionnaire will still feel uncomfortable and will choose not to disclose any information on their sexual attraction to children, so the rate of around one in five men is likely to be a minimum figure.

There are far fewer data on women than on men paedophiles. It is suggested that adult sexual behaviour with children involves men rather than women 'by a ratio of approximately 10:1' (Feierman 1990: 10), possibly because of the neurochemical processes of embryonic masculinisation and defeminisation referred to earlier.

What can we learn from these studies? The most important point is that attempting to learn about adult sexual attraction to children by studying only samples of known sex offenders is pretty likely to give a distorted picture (Cossins 1999, 2000). As Finkelhor and colleagues pointed out some while ago now, it is only those men who have been unlucky enough to be caught, and inarticulate enough not to persuade the authorities to let them off, who end up as known sex offenders (Finkelhor *et al.* 1986). Given the conviction rates in England and Wales, for example, as discussed earlier, it seems fairly plausible that most men sexually attracted to children, including those who go on to have direct sexual contact with children, are not in prison but out in the community – and it is in the community that we must find them and learn about their experiences. The following chapter begins this process by providing an introduction to the 'online paedophile community'.

2   Paedophiles online

Introduction

Up until a few years ago, the only sources of information available to those attempting to understand adult sexual attraction to children were dusty medical tomes or sensationalised tabloid reports. Today we have the Internet, and this has revolutionised how we can now go about looking for information, and the sorts of information we can find. Most significantly, the Internet has broken down geographical barriers. The physical location of a person, or a computer, becomes, on the Internet, both unknown and irrelevant.

Of the approximately 2 billion people on Earth who are able to communicate in some form of English, there are 380 million who use English to communicate on the Internet. English is the most popular Internet language, with just over 30 per cent of all online communication now conducted in English (Internet World Stats 2007). The disappearance of geographical barriers, together with the prevalence of English as a global language, means that it now matters very little whether I am physically based in Australia, Canada, Britain, the Indian subcontinent, Ireland, New Zealand, southern Africa, the USA, the West Indies, or any of a huge number of other countries: provided I can access the Internet and communicate in basic written English, the same information will be available for me to access wherever I live and, in turn, the information I choose to post on the Internet can be accessed and can influence the beliefs and the behaviour of, potentially, millions of other people. There are therefore no longer any effective barriers or boundaries to the spread of information, for good or for ill.

This chapter is divided into three sections, each dealing with a specific aspect of the online experience. Section I examines file-sharing in the 'Darknet' and how people may guard their online privacy. Section II is specifically about sharing child pornography and other forms of graphic art which portray young children sexually, while Section III is concerned with legal and visible aspects of the 'online paedophile community'. Information on the Internet, provided by a mere handful of individuals, is potentially capable of affecting the views of literally millions of people, and so this chapter ends with a brief examination of the ways in which pro-paedophile arguments are presented and contested online. Later on, in the chapters dealing with paedophiles' own experiences, this book explores in more detail the ways in which the Internet is used as an 'online community'.

Section I: Spiders in the Darknet

A key function of cyberspace is to facilitate sharing, and in particular the sharing of files, whether those are software, photographs, audio or music files or film. Sharing is at the very heart of the original dream of the Internet. Web-programmers have, essentially, two visions of what they are doing. The first is a revolutionary utopian vision of the unfettered distribution of non-copyrighted, free to use, 'open source freeware' or 'shareware' software codes, with individuals working collaboratively and creatively together to build something bigger and braver and more democratic than anything humans could possibly have previously achieved: this is the vision of Jimbo Wales of Wikipedia, for example, or of the collaborative SETI (Search for Extra-Terrestrial Intelligence, a scientific project based at the University of California, Berkeley) or climate-change projects taking place across millions of individual PCs. The second vision, originally a minority view, is a concept of the web as a place to make money, exemplified by Bill Gates' Microsoft corporation. Making money – capitalism – requires control of resources, otherwise people will simply take without paying. These two visions have, so far, clashed most sharply and publicly over the issue of music downloads. Underlying these two opposing visions is the original function of the Internet in its first incarnation as the ARPANET, a military technology, with its focus on secure information-transmission, the building of 'firewalls' to resist infiltration and network-survivability in the face of attack. Particularly since 9/11, a felt need for greater (governmental) surveillance and control over what information is on the Internet runs alongside a felt need for greater (individual) privacy and evasion of control. Within this convoluted context, how it is practically possible for people to share files?

File-sharing as a huge Internet phenomenon began in 1999 with Napster, a software programme to seek out and download music files. The Napster software was free to download – and suddenly, peer-to-peer file-sharing meant that anyone could access any music, regardless of copyright. Napster was quickly prosecuted, but after Napster came more sophisticated systems such as Gnutella. This makes use of members' personal computer hard-drives to store and transmit files, and thus it becomes almost impossible to know who has sent or who has received any particular file. The next step on from Gnutella is Freenet. Freenet is a P2P (peer-to-peer) system which was set up by its originator, Ian Clark, quite specifically and deliberately to counter any form of online censorship. A decentralised system like Gnutella, Freenet also employs encryption, with all files that are transmitted being put into formats that resist 'traffic sniffing' or finding out what is being sent. Anyone can publish information easily, without having to buy a domain-name as they would when posting files on a website. While file-sharing started off as an activity that occurred typically between friends or at least people socially connected to each other, in a system such as Freenet people will have no idea who they are sharing files with, or where in the world the file may be coming from. File-sharing may thus take place in a huge anonymous virtual space, inhabited by tens of thousands of individuals.

Since the World Wide Web contains billions of web pages, it would be physically impossible for any individual to sift through them to locate specific information. Therefore search engines have been developed to do this. Search engines use special software called 'spiders' which roam around the web, automatically following hyperlinks from one document to the next and extracting important textual information from them which search engines then use to build up a huge index correlating keywords to web pages. This information is stored in a database, ready to be accessed when a user types a query into the search engine. Google, for example, now claims to have over 2 billion pages in its database. However, a very large portion of the web is completely invisible to spiders. This is partly because search engines are searching a saved database rather than the live web, where content changes and increases constantly, but it is also because some sites are deliberately set up to be unsearchable by spiders. For example, with Freenet, since it is not part of the Internet, its pages are not searchable by search engines such as Google and are therefore invisible to all outside the Freenet community. Parts of the Internet such as these, which are not accessible to the general public, are known as the 'Darknet'.

Freenet is a particularly interesting example of the 'Darknet' because it is so explicit about its high-minded philosophy of free speech and protection of democracy, while conspicuously ignoring the reality that it serves as a major haven for child pornographers. On its main pages, Freenet's founder, Ian Clark, expounds his philosophy which includes the following statements:

> Freedom of speech, in most western cultures, is generally considered to be one of the most important rights any individual might have. ... It is standard practice for most western governments to lie to their populations, so much so, that people now take it for granted, despite the fact that this undermines the very democratic principles which justify the government's existence in the first place. ... The only way to ensure that a democracy will remain effective is to ensure that the government cannot control its population's ability to share information, to communicate. So long as everything we see and hear is filtered, we are not truly free. Freenet's aim is to allow two or more people who wish to share information, to do so.
>
> (Clark 2008)

To discuss (and refute) censorship, Clark uses the example of racism. To defend the policy of anonymity, Clark claims, 'You cannot have freedom of speech without the option to remain anonymous. Most censorship is retrospective, it is generally much easier to curtail free speech by punishing those who exercise it afterward, rather than preventing them from doing it in the first place. The only way to prevent this is to remain anonymous.' Clark also explains that, because enforcement of copyright requires monitoring of communications, therefore 'Freenet, a system designed to protect Freedom of Speech, must prevent enforcement of copyright.' Having set out his claims for freedom of speech as a good which overrules many other goods (such as the good of preventing racist speech or the good of not stealing), Clark then defines Freenet:

> Freenet is free software which lets you publish and obtain information on the Internet without fear of censorship. ... Without anonymity there can never be true freedom of speech, and without decentralization the network will be vulnerable to attack. Communications by Freenet nodes are encrypted and are 'routed-through' other nodes to make it extremely difficult to determine who is requesting the information and what its content is. Users contribute to the network by giving bandwidth and a portion of their hard drive (called the 'data store') for storing files. Unlike other peer-to-peer file sharing networks, Freenet does not let the user control what is stored in the data store. Instead, files are kept or deleted depending on how popular they are, with the least popular being discarded to make way for newer or more popular content. Files in the data store are encrypted to reduce the likelihood of prosecution by persons wishing to censor Freenet content.

The Freenet developers apparently continue to assume, idealistically, that their site defends free speech. However, commentators, for example on Slashdot.org (a website for computer programmers, accessed February 2008) are dubious, pointing out that 'Free speech is founded not only on the protection of individual freedom, but also on accountability; you must take responsibility for what you say' and that 'Freenet's not about peddling your thoughts and speeches. It's about peddling kiddie porn and MP3s.' Similarly, despite their claims to protect global democracy, it is in fact only in the Western world, where democracy is not under significant threat, that the necessary infrastructure exists to support Freenet (for example, thousands of homes with stable connections to the Internet). In underdeveloped countries, where democracy is often genuinely under threat, the conditions to support the use of Freenet do not actually exist. Again, although Clark suggests that Freenet can defend democracy by providing a platform where disparate views can be aired and understood, it seems more likely that it actually functions to support small subcultures who talk only among themselves, thereby embedding their own worldviews more deeply. As one commentator states (on Global Ideas Bank 2008), 'There are numerous documents on Freenet that allude to child pornography. ... These documents are not open discussion, rather sites created by and for the community they allude to. Rather than trying to unite people of opposing views, Freenet links together the people of their own type with each other.' In fact, far from Freenet being the web's only home for vigorous political debate, there is almost certainly vastly more political debate held quite openly on the Internet, leaving Freenet and other parts of the 'Darknet' as, *de facto,* the only sites on the web where child pornography, not high-minded political debate, can be published.

So far, Freenet has been downloaded by over 2 million users, but this hardly compares with the popularity of mainstream P2P music-sharing sites which typically have users numbering in the tens of millions and above. This makes it quite a specialist market, serving only a tiny proportion of the total web population, presumably including those with most to hide. Freenet resists censorship in a number of ways, including the ironic fact that, if authorities were to request a file from a node, they would get a copy but it would be impossible for them to prove that the file was there before they requested it, thus leaving them open to counter-claims of entrapment. Also, as the files are encrypted when stored, the node owner can plausibly deny any knowledge that the file was there. Finally, rather than removing offending files, each request by censors would have the self-defeating effect of generating new copies of that file on the Freenet network. More recently, Freenet has increased its security yet again. In 2006, a new version, Freenet 0.7, was released, using a 'scalable darknet' architecture, where security is increased by allowing users to limit which other peers their peer will communicate with directly. As they state, 'This means that not only does Freenet aim to prevent others from finding out what you are doing with Freenet, it makes it extremely difficult for them to even know that you are running a Freenet node at all' (information from Freenet site, accessed 15 February 2008). Who on the web requires such extreme security?

Section II: Child pornography

Supporters of anti-censorship sites such as Freenet often use a 1996 quotation from the cyber-rights campaigner and Wikipedia consultant lawyer, Mike Godwin:

> I worry about my child and the Internet all the time, even though she's too young to have logged on yet. Here's what I worry about. I worry that 10 or 15 years from now, she will come to me and say 'Daddy, where were you when they took freedom of the press away from the Internet?'
> (Quoted, for example, on http://freenetproject.org/)

Other individuals have more immediate worries about children. One unpublished 2005 study by a student in the Netherlands, Koen Leurs, found a thriving paedophile community utilising Freenet. Leurs found, 'The lack of censorship that characterises Freenet, paved the way for child lovers to speak freely about their motivations' (2005: 25). To support his claims, Leurs provides the example of the following conversation, posted on a message board between 23 October and 19 December 2004:

BlackMidnight@LsBX13QAfeLQVIFhFHTCPof1eSE – 2004.10.23 –
18:34:10GMT –

Answer truthfully, there is no reason to lie. Do you have sex with preteen
girls and boys?

Me first: No I dont.

—zargon 10@xiCUNVtDoG30WrwqKkvZOIKVNcI – 2004.10.23 –
21:17:18GMT –

No, I don't and won't. But they can be cute…

—Anonymous – 2004.11.01 – 23:51:31GMT –

not yet.

—Anonymous – 2004.11.14 – 15:21:34GMT –

Once had some touching and licking, more than 10 yrs ago, nothing since.

—Anonymous – 2004.12.19 – 11:15:23GMT –

I did some touching and licking of a babygirl when she was between 5
months and her first birthday. That was 2 years ago, she was my first and
I did not do any ever since. (Her parents moved away, maybe better this way.)

He also gives an example of comment posted on a 'freesite' (Freenet website)
edited by someone called Napthala, inviting responses on Freenet boards:

How would you react if you get asked by a 12 yo boy if you would suck him?
Well I would get red in that case…would it be wrong to do what he likes?
what he askes you? Don't you think it was hard enough to ask? […] Dont be
shy, ask me on frost, tell me what you think, (boards: cl, freenet, frost)

People could not only speak freely but also share child pornography files.
Information about which files are available, and the content of files, is shared on
message boards, particularly private message boards created within Frost (a file-
sharing and messaging programme within Freenet). Within the comments and
signatures posted on these messages boards, links are provided to 'freesites' (the
Freenet equivalent of websites) that are otherwise invisible and unlocatable.
Since freesites are not indexed, there are no search engines which could find
them. The freesites therefore provide individuals with private spaces where child
pornography can be uploaded and distributed. Leurs refers to Frost being
known as 'the largest online child pornography-oriented videotheque' and provides an example of a transaction using Frost:

—guantanamo@Rmuj1hotSZM3ZtKKJ4XfLdfg+qY – 2005.05.23 –
12:20:10GMT –

Hi, could anyone post a key list of the fantastic series 'lolitas desire'? It
would be lovable thank you

—ntwrk@ty35jr9P+m7+bw2kr0terV6vqgQ   –   2005.05.30   –
12:26:00GMT –

Here is one for you.

CHK@shou3uBXZgd~jzDzL78kjPZHmVwOAwI,owma7M17u-
dUJzeCKr5HXbQ/suniy.rar

(preteen-board)

As Leurs demonstrates, and as Jenkins found in his earlier (2001) study of bulletin boards and newsgroups, the sharing of such files takes place within a surprisingly chatty environment, where there seems to be a strongly felt need, at least among some participants, to justify, negotiate, minimise, deny, confront or otherwise come to terms with the illegal, socially condemned and highly disturbing material they are accessing, collecting and masturbating to – material which provides graphic visual evidence of the psychological destruction of the young children involved.

Much of the material circulating on the Internet appears to be very recent. This is because of two factors. One is that the market appears to be expanding, thus creating constant demand for more material. The other is that child pornography as a mass phenomenon is actually still fairly new. Published commercial child pornography hardly existed until 1969, when the general liberalisation of attitudes in Scandinavia and the Netherlands resulted in the production of many magazines and films catering to paedophile interests and available through sex shops or mail-order catalogues. However, by around 1979 this market had effectively been stopped and from the early 1980s there was virtually no child pornography available for purchase and almost zero quantities of new material being produced. As Jenkins states (2001: 40), by the mid-1980s 'the whole business appeared to be on the verge of extinction'. New technologies such as videos did not significantly alter the situation, as sending them through the post could result in arrest and a link back to the distributors and producers. It was only the development of online bulletin boards (BBSs) and newsgroups in the 1980s that rescued and revived the market for child pornography. The first child-pornography BBSs probably began by 1982, taking advantage of the ability to distribute material outside the postal system, and also of the ambiguous extra-territorial legal situation existing when images are circulated across national borders and differing jurisdictions. 'Already by the late 1980s', suggests Jenkins, 'pedophiles and child pornography enthusiasts were among the most experienced and knowledgeable members of the computerised communication world' (2001: 47), far ahead of others including law enforcement officers. And, as he points out, 'There are today veterans whose careers in circulating electronic child porn span twenty years or more' (2001: 48). Thus child pornographers have embedded themselves firmly into the fabric of the web and have built up expertise in this area which very few police agencies can match.

With the development of the technologies of CD-burning, web-cameras, VOIP ('voice over Internet protocol' such as Skype), MP4 and MPEG4 video-streaming software, and the capacity for Internet connection and video-recording by mobile phone (cell-phone), the processes of child pornography manufacture and distribution are doubtless shifting again. But it seems unlikely that, with Freenet continuing to offer such a congenial climate, child-pornography distributors would yet feel any need to stray far from its welcoming embrace.

Since Jenkins wrote, new technologies such as BitTorrent have made the downloading of large files, such as films, even easier and quicker. BitTorrent is a form of P2P file-sharing which distributes large amounts of data widely across a number of computers in a system known as 'swarming'. It was designed by Bram Cohen in 2001 and became popular immediately, despite concerns over the illegal distribution of copyright material. By 2004 it was claimed by British web analysis firm CacheLogic (Pasick 2004) that BitTorrent accounted for a massive 35 per cent of all traffic on the Internet, more than all other P2P programs combined, and dwarfing mainstream traffic such as webpages. Even a quick glimpse at a BitTorrent website such as Torrent.ffnn. nl (accessed 17 February 2008) throws up files with the names, '7yo Jackie', 'naked preteen girls pictures' and 'lolicom'.

Much child pornography featuring underage girls is known by terms derived from the word 'lolita'. The name Lolita was the invented pet name given by the narrator, Humbert Humbert, to the twelve-year-old girl Dolores Haze in the book *Lolita* by Vladimir Nabokov, first published in 1955. Since the publication of the book (and two films of the same name), this name has become a common international code word to relate to sexuality in relation to underage girls. Jenkins found that the men exchanging child pornography on bulletin boards and newsgroups often described themselves as 'loli-lovers'. The word Lolita has also given rise to the term 'Lolita complex' which is used to refer to a particular type within the form of graphic Japanese art known as manga (cartoons or comics) and anime (animated cartoons). If you are not familiar with manga and anime characters, think of the human figures in the enormously popular Pokemon or Digimon series, with their strange, almost square, eyes and stylised (often spiky and pastel-coloured) hair. 'Lolita complex' cartoons feature schoolgirls or younger girls, often explicitly sexualised. These combine saccharine cuteness and innocence (huge eyes, lots of teddybears) with both clearly pornographic sexual explicitness and at times with violence. The cartoon style has also spawned a real-life fashion style, known as Elegant Gothic Lolita, worn by teenage or young adult women in Japan. It has also influenced mainstream girls' dolls and cartoons, such as the Bratz, Bratz Kidz and Bratz Babies characters, who again combine traits of extreme infantilisation such as disproportionately large heads and eyes, very small noses (and chubby legs and the use of baby-bottles among the Bratz Babies), with precocious sexualisation such as the portrayal of adult-proportioned breasts, waists and hips among the Bratz, disproportionately long legs, and interests centred on a consuming 'passion for fashion' and the kind of pop music popularised by the Spice Girls.

In manga or anime, the term 'Lolita complex' is generally shortened to 'lolicom', 'lolicon', 'lolikon' or other transliterations from the Japanese such as 'rorikon'. The male equivalent, relating to young boys, is termed 'shota', 'shotacon', 'shotakon', or 'syotacon'. The term 'lolicon', as well as referring to images, also refers to the enthusiasts or fans of lolicon, who often obsessively amass large collections of manga, anime, dolls and figurines of lolicon cartoon characters.

Some sites dealing with lolicon or shotacon are clearly dealing in pornographic imagery featuring extremely graphic representations of children engaged in sexual acts. Lolicon has a strong web presence and even a very cursory search of the web using a search engine such as Google is likely to produce a range of cartoon images which range from the bland to the bizarre and the extremely pornographic, with websites which carry no 'adult' warning but which show, on their home-page, very graphic and disturbing cartoon-images. Bizarrely, viewing and collecting lolicon seems to have become a subcultural norm, especially in Japan, a medium through which disaffected men may choose to express their sense of anomie and disconnection with society. One cultural critic, Hiroki Azuma, suggests that: 'For [people] who feel at odds with society, or are excluded from society, pedophilic manga is the most convenient [form of rebellion]. ... Even people who have absolutely no interest in pedophilia, begin to feel as if they are the sort of "no good" person who should be attracted to little girls' (quoted in McNicol 2004).

The issue of images which do not involve real children but which portray 'virtual' images representing child pornography is a vexed question which has proved difficult for legislators in a number of countries. In the USA, in 2002, the Supreme Court struck down a six-year-old law banning virtual child pornography and established a subsequent Child Obscenity and Pornography Prevention Act which banned only those virtual images which are indistinguishable from real child pornography, and also prohibited all obscene pornographic images of prepubescent children. However, such images are not illegal or considered socially taboo in Japanese culture, although this appears possibly to be changing. Growing concerns have been reported over lolicon recently after the kidnapping and murder of a small girl by a man obsessed with lolicon images (Anime News Network 2005). More recently, one lolicon enthusiast wondered on his blog about the relationship between looking at lolicon and finding children in real life sexually attractive. In his article, 'Are you an anime-lolicon that could turn into a RL-pedo?', he mused,

> Is it really ok to continue raving about these underaged anime beauties? What if the 2D obsession literally takes an extra dimension? Thankfully, after much reflection on my interaction with RL [real-life] girls of ages 7 to 17 yrs. I came to the conclusion that even if I could be classified as a type of anime lolicon, it'd NEVER translate into RL pedophilia. This is predicated on the belief that the anime lolis I like DO NOT EXIST in RL.
>
> ('Stripey' 2007)

Other examples of online obsessions that hover uncomfortably close to actual child pornography are 'doll albums', in which cartoon images of girls, or actual plastic models of girls, can be 'dressed up'. In The Doll Palace (www. thedollpalace.com/doll-maker/dress-up-games.php), manga-style cartoon figures are presented, and the viewer can select clothes, hair and so forth to 'display' their 'doll' in an 'album'. The figures are displayed in a range of styles, which include 'Lolita' and 'Glamour'. This site is owned by 'Jessica' or 'Jezz' who describes 'herself' as aged nineteen. In one section of the website,

'Jezz' writes 'Stories for Kids', which are commented on by people signing themselves with names such as 'Dadezgurl' and 'AngelaPRETTY', with given ages ranging from thirteen to nineteen, all of which seems rather unlikely for an activity of this sort. One hopes that actual small girls do not stumble upon this site by accident. A much more explicitly pornographic example of this hobby is provided at Dollalbum.com which contains an 'adult' warning before entering and which shows figures which are basically plastic sex dolls dressed up, posed, photographed and then adjusted in Photoshop to make them look as lifelike as possible. As Leurs (2005) has pointed out, within these areas of online fantasy erotica (which are presumably legal), it is a small step to digitally construct pornographic images which would presumably be not only illegal but which would carry severe penalties (at least in some jurisdictions) to download.

Section III: Online advocacy and online attack

[I] looked up [some information] on Wikipedia, and from there found the 'Pedophile Activism' page. This was I think my first experience with that concept. ... Later on I returned to this article by myself. The page about Alice Day that Wikipedia linked to was on Puellula. ... Over time, I returned to those pages repeatedly, reading more about the pedophile activism of the past and learning about the life and views of the owner of Puellula. Many of the things that were said made a great deal of sense to me. I did a lot of thinking about the subject, but I also did a lot of what could be considered compulsive reading of these sites – it made me feel better just to know there were others like me out there, and I wanted to get that feeling as often as I could. I visited many of the sites linked to by Puellula, as well as some others linked to from Wikipedia.

(Kristof)

[T]he reason I spend so much time at Wikipedia is that their Paedophilia article is the top result for that term on Google, making it an important platform for us.

('BLueRibbon')

The previous section has demonstrated that Freenet and other P2P file-sharing sites are clearly of central importance in distributing child pornography, and the sites (both commercial and amateur) for lolicon and shotacon anime and other forms of 'virtual' child pornography are also highly significant in catering to the tastes of those who find sexualised images of children erotically attractive. However, these are not the only and perhaps not even the most important ways in which adult sexual attraction to children is mediated in cyberspace. What may be of more significance are the legal and easily accessible sites where paedophilia as a lived experience, philosophy or lifestyle choice can be discussed and advocated for. These sites have included, for example, Puellula and The Human Face of Pedophilia, both set up and run by the activist Lindsay Ashford and both closed down in 2007. Such sites have now become the main place where paedophiles speak to one another and to the wider world about what adult sexual attraction is and what it means. Before the Internet, such conversations might have been limited only to obscure underground journals: now they potentially reach tens of millions of people (Goode 2008a; 2008b). In 1995 the sociologist Ken Plummer discussed the hidden and silent nature of the 'sexual stories' told by paedophiles. As he described it, these stories are

> on a spectrum which is arrayed from the conservative to the radical. Some speak in Boy Scout Leader tones about the purity of the man–boy relationship and whose stories provide manuals of etiquette for behaviour between adult and child. Others see the adult–child relationship as a revolutionary act. A paedophile who enters this world has an array of stories that can be drawn upon in making sense of the experience.
>
> (Plummer 1995: 118)

This spectrum of stories is now increasingly available online. Any understanding of contemporary paedophilia must take full cognisance of the constantly changing and complex cultural world of the 'online paedophile community' as it provides discussion, debate, support and advocacy for English-speaking paedophiles around the globe – and is in its turn contested and attacked by the online anti-paedophile community.

In the following chapter, in the discussion on how the Minor-Attracted Adults (MAA) Daily Lives Research Project originated, I will introduce a 'thought experiment' on what someone might do if they began to be worried about their own feelings of sexual attraction to children. Suffice it to say here that, as the world becomes increasingly used to turning to the Internet for information, for many people the most likely place to search for information on any topic will typically be the search engine Google and, through Google, pages from the online encyclopedia Wikipedia. Links from Wikipedia articles can then take the searcher directly to websites, like Puellula and its newer incarnations, which specifically advocate for a positive self-identity for adults sexually attracted to children. These websites form the basis of the 'online paedophile community', and their impact is explored in some depth in the following chapters on the findings from the MAA Daily Lives Research Project. Before we turn to those, however, it is important in this section to spend a little time examining the process by which most individuals will find such websites for the first time, which is likely to be through search engines and through Wikipedia. Wikipedia is thus a major clearing house of information on paedophilia, as on so much else, on the Internet.

The significance of Wikipedia as a 'first port of call' for information on paedophilia has not gone unnoticed by the online paedophile community – nor, indeed, by the online anti-paedophile community: the following quotations are taken from the 'Wikipedia Campaign' page at the anti-paedophile activist Wikisposure.com website. One pro-paedophile activist, BLue-Ribbon, explains, 'the reason I spend so much time at Wikipedia is that their Paedophilia article is the top result for that term on Google, making it an important platform for us'. Another poster, Student, comments, on the topic of whether one should declare oneself as a paedophile on the editors' 'user pages':

> Let's be pragmatic, here.
>
> The most important function wikipedia serves is via the pedophilia articles themselves. It is important that they remain fair and unbiased. It is important that they continue to have external links to the support and activist community. The user pages are much less important.
>
> It is of the utmost importance that pedophiles newly daring to google 'pedophile' or 'pedophilia', or look them up directly in wikipedia, in an effort to understand themselves better, are able to get unbiased information and are presented with links to a support forum like GC and/or sites like Lindsay's human face of pedophilia. Many of these men and women are in dire need of support.
>
> Secondly, nonpedophiles who recognise the increasingly sensationalistic media treatment, etc., and turn to the web to find the facts or people who use the web as their primary source of information: If they turn to wikipedia, wikipedia should give a fair and balanced view. This community needs that to happen. Wikipedia provides the opportunity for a widely recognised channel to fairly present the story. This community must do what it can to keep that channel open. And again, we need to keep the links in that article as well.
>
> That should be the primary focus of our wikipedia efforts. If you have to 'lie and hide' to keep our influence balanced against the bigots, then by all means lie and hide to do it. By all means, do not give up the fight to self-identify on the user pages, but make sure you do not let it stop you from editing!
>
> (quoted on Wikisposure website 2008)

Information dissemination on the Internet has evolved into a very subtle game, aided by the anonymity which posters such as 'Student' can deliberately foster. Both paedophiles and 'antis' infiltrate and attempt to control one another's sites in various ways. Anti-paedophile activists, for example, take down paedophile sites and represent them under the old name but with hostile new messages (see, for example, sites such as 'Human Face of Pedophilia Blogspot'). Both 'peds' and 'antis' also appear to operate as trolls, deliberately posting inflammatory remarks to provoke others into responding. They may also operate as 'concern trolls', posing as supporters of a particular view but subtly sowing concerns which undermine their opponents' activities (Moulitsas 2008). Information on the Internet, therefore, may be posted to provide straightforward information, to challenge and question, to irritate, to sow seeds of doubt, or to deliberately misinform. There are many articles within the Wikipedia site, constantly changing, which relate to the topic of paedophilia and in which this process of information and disinformation can be scrutinised. An in-depth examination of the process of using Wikipedia articles to disseminate and contest pro-paedophile positions, using the specific example of the definition of 'child grooming', is presented in Goode (forthcoming).

Over the short period from around late 2005 to late 2007, there was a particular flurry of activity documented on Wikipedia and other sites, as the opportunity to present, defend, debate and challenge pro-paedophile views was recognised and vigorously seized. The neutrality and objectivity of Wikipedia was challenged, for example, by the activist Daniel Brandt on his website Wikipedia-Watch. org., but by December 2005 a claim was being made about Wikipedia editors which was significantly more detailed and forceful. The Wikipedophilia debate began on 12 December 2005 with a posting purporting to be from an organisation called Parents for the Online Safety of Children (POSC). The posting was sent to Perverted-Justice.com who published it (Perverted Justice are an anti-paedophile activist group perhaps most well known for arranging the sting operations broadcast on the US television series *To Catch a Predator*). The posting was headed 'Online Encyclopedia is a Gathering for Internet Predators: WHO IS EDITING THE INTERNET'S ENCYCLOPEDIA?' The text of the article read:

> Wikipedia.com: you can find links to it everywhere. Online forums, scholarly journals, blogs, high school research papers. Wikipedia is an 'open source' encyclopedia with the philosophy of democratic contribution. This encyclopedia differs from other more established encyclopedias by its editors; Wikipedia is composed of anonymous people contributing, deleting, and voting on various aspects of articles. Wikipedia is the frontier of online information distribution, with over 830,000 articles in the English language.
>
> It does have many criticisms, but there is one very important question that goes ignored by the mainstream media and wikifans alike. Who, exactly, edits wikipedia?
>
> It has come to the attention of the Parents for the Online Safety of Children (POSC) that there is a underground cabal of pedophiles who edit wikipedia, trying to make wikipedia a distribution center for pedophile propaganda.

The posting continued by naming a number of editors, of whom four – Zanthalon, identified as Lindsay Ashford or David Alway (Zanthalon blogspot 2007), LuxOfTKGL, identified as Darren Cresswell (Human Face of Pedophilia Blogspot 2008), Clayboy and Rookiee, identified as Damien Cole (Mountaineer 2007) – are self-defined paedophiles. In addition, three other editors were named in a context which suggested they might be paedophile or pro-paedophile, and the posting continued with the suggestion:

Since wikipedia allows pedophiles to edit wikipedia pages and view the IP addresses of children freely, we recommend that you use filtering software to block wikipedia from access in your household or school. ... Since wikipedia refuses to address the issue of pedophiles within its ranks and the allowance of random editing to pages, we can only recommend parents to withhold access to wikipedia.com for the time being.

Perverted Justice commented on this posting (emphases and ellipses in original):

[W]e ourselves know how organized online pedophiles are. It's hardly shocking to us that a ring of pedophiles has concentrated itself on Wikipedia, it's just shocking that Wikipedia seems just fine with this development. ... It is disgraceful that Wikipedia would allow pedophiles to edit entries on pedophiles...not simply because they're pedophiles (*though that should be enough of a reason to disallow them*) but also because each Wikipedia article is supposed to be NPOV. Neutral Point of View. Pedophiles do not have a Neutral Point of View, and the fact that they're allowed...and *encouraged* by those elevated to Wikipedia administration just illustrates yet another failing of the Wiki ideal. We echo the call for Parents to block Wikipedia from their child's research resources until they implement a better system of authoring.

On behalf of Wikipedia, a Wikipedia administrator named Linuxbeak (Alex Schenck) then responded (and a fuller and more detailed response is also available at http://en.wikipedia.org/wiki/User: Linuxbeak/Angry_letter, dated 13 December 2005):

It is not Wikipedia's goal to promote any one said stance, nor is it our goal to serve as a basis for propaganda. We strive to be as neutral and unbiased as possible.

Concerns have been raised in the past regarding neutrality of topics. This press release is obviously critical of how we allow alleged pedophiles to edit articles on pedophilia to the extent of allowing them to push an agenda of pro-pedophilia. To this concern, we do not have any major objections. Pedophilia is one of our less-monitored articles, and it has been pointed out that there are a number of editors who have declared themselves pedophiles who also actively edit pedophilia-related articles. This brings up three issues.

First: Wikipedia and the Wikimedia Foundation does *not* endorse any type of illegal activity, including sexual activity with a child or person that is under the age of consent. Wikipedia will not tolerate child-grooming or 'fishing', and those who do this and are caught will be banned as well as information being handed over to the proper authorities.

Second: Wikipedia's policy to maintain a neutral point of view is not so much an end as it is a path. Certain articles such as pedophilia must be pointed out and identified as being of a non-neutral point of view, and as such fixed to be such. This does not mean, however, that we will tolerate an anti-pedophilia point of view to an article, just as much as we will not tolerate a pro-pedophilia point of view. The point of an encyclopedia is to provide facts. To this, we pledge that we will strive to do just that.

Third: Although this is only conjecture, the majority of humanity finds pedophilia to be taboo and/or immoral. With that said, Wikipedia and the Wikimedia Foundation are not responsible for the viewpoints of individuals which use its services and resources. It is not our job to tell our users what is right and what is wrong; instead it is our job as administrators and editors to ensure that nothing illegal is being committed, which includes trolling for children. As previously stated, we will not tolerate illegal activity.

In the sense used here, 'trolling' would mean browsing, lurking or deliberately 'baiting' a post and waiting for someone (in this case, a child) to respond, much like putting a baited line in the water and waiting for a fish to bite (Donath 1999). Meanwhile, the POSC posting appeared on a new site, Wikipedophilia, launched on 13 December 2005, with the strap-line 'News and analysis of Wikipedia's anti-child practices' and the text:

Wikipedophilia.com has launched to provide news and analysis of the latest controversy surrounding Wikipedia; the harboring and support of an active community of pro-pedophilia contributors and moderators. We are here to provide you with timely information regarding the status of the pedophilia related entries on Wikipedia, as well as any steps, or lack thereof, taken by Wikipedia in the matter. The discloser of sexual predators within the Wikipedia ranks [is an example] of Wikipedia's systemic problem of content inaccuracy and their continuing protection of dangerous persons under the banner of 'anonymity'. Protect your children, block Wikipedia!

This website appears to have lasted only two months, since no new postings are given after January 2006, but in June 2007 the founder of Perverted Justice, Xavier von Erck (also known as Phillip John Eide, for example see Corrupted-Justice 2005) set up the Wikisposure website to investigate paedophile activists posting on Wikipedia and other sites.

An alternative point of view to those expressed by POSC, Perverted Justice and Wikipedophilia is that given by Clayboy, a self-defined paedophile referred to earlier, and an editor for Wikipedia. The following material is taken from the (now-defunct) Clayboy user page (http://en.wikipedia.org/wiki/User: Clayboy, accessed 4 June 2006). Clayboy had tried to post an article on the term 'Boylover', and states:

To most people, the subject alone is outrageous, it is unthinkable, the very idea is so thoroughly filthy they get an urge to shower immediately.

If you knew me, you would probably feel the same about me. ... [I love boys but] my firm convictions tell me I would sooner chew my hand off than even consider anything sexual with a boy. ... You are still free to gag and vomit at the idea of me, and most people would. ... We are simply social outcasts because a part of what we are triggers a moral outrage. ... The truth about us cannot be written down in a collaborative medium such as Wikipedia. Everybody 'knows' everything about us already, and if we attempt to share a truth, which we can only do anonymously online, that truth is not compatible with what 99.9 percent of the rest of Wikipedia already 'know' about us. We simply cannot compete with the sheer man-power. In a subject so ultimately taboo, truths cannot survive, so any article about the subject is not of an encyclopedic nature and can best be seen as a documentary of prejudice and oppression. I will continue to try to keep the worst lies out of the articles, but I know that in the long run, the case is lost.

This emotional outpouring does seem to sit oddly with what others might regard as the undue stress on pro-paedophile material already existing in Wikipedia. When it is compared, for example, to the 2006 biography of Benjamin Britten, *Britten's Children* (Bridcut 2006), including discussion of his well-documented attraction to pre-pubescent boys (Mars-Jones 2006) then it is clear that, to 'most people' the subject is far from 'unthinkable' or 'ultimately taboo', but is in fact becoming acknowledged as a facet of the lives of certain individuals.

While Wikipedia has been challenged as containing an 'underground cabal of pedophiles' who unduly influence the editorial process, the reality appears to be somewhat different, with a large number of contributors being involved in a generally considerate and thoughtful online discussion to develop a col-laborative consensus on aspects of knowledge. Clearly, self-defined paedo-philes were found who are involved in the process of editing, but this is perhaps not surprising given the demographics of Wikipedia contributors, including the very high proportion of men. Since being challenged by anti-paedophile activists such as Perverted Justice, various changes have taken place at Wikipedia. For example, Rookiee's user page was taken down and he was blocked on 21 September 2006 for using his page for advocacy; the user-page of LuxOfTKGL seems to have been unused since 26 September 2006; Clayboy's user page was taken down on 7 March 2007 for 'activity detri-mental to the activity of Wikipedia'; and an arbitration case was filed against Zanthalon on 15 March 2007. These actions have removed four of the most outspoken pro-paedophile activists who were editing Wikipedia (although it appears BLueRibbon, Student and other activists are quietly stepping into the breach). In addition, anti-paedophile activists have edited new articles for Wikipedia, on 'anti-paedophile activism' and other topics, to counter the pro-paedophile articles still extant. However, Xavier von Erck (as username XavierVE), the founder of Perverted Justice, in a curious twist, has himself now been blocked, apparently for too many contentious edits: his user page has been blocked as from 4 March 2008.

Thus, as this section documents, both pro-paedophile advocacy and anti-paedophile attack of such advocacy are widely available and easily found on the Internet, not merely in the furtive and encrypted underworld of the 'Darknet' but rather in full view on Wikipedia, one of the most popular and frequently visited websites in all cyberspace.

3 Setting up the Minor-Attracted Adults Daily Lives Project

*The secret shame of paedophilia is a pervasively crippling experience, and it does not just make a person feel broken and divided, it makes them act that way. ... I saw absolutely no alternative but to keep my thoughts and feelings shut away in a dark little closet. I felt my life would be over if I ever shared my secret with **anyone**, and I was very afraid that one day I would be 'found out'. That was a terrible way to live, as you might imagine. I'm sure I'm a much more balanced and self disciplined person now that I do speak to a few people about it, and this effect could only be enhanced if my acceptance were more tangible and complete.*

(Tim)

Introduction

Up to this point, this book has dealt with information which is entirely in the public domain and can be found by anyone with a library subscription and an Internet account. This part of the book now deals with original research which I undertook between 2006 and 2008 to explore the everyday experiences and views of 'minor-attracted adults' (MAAs) themselves.

The previous chapters of the book have indicated something of the current situation and some of the problems that arise from this situation. But the perspective so far has tended to be 'from the outside', trying to make sense of how we as a society view paedophilia and adult sexual contact with children. This is a limited perspective in that much remains unknown. Most scientific studies on paedophiles to date have made use of samples drawn from those who have been convicted of offences, or who have entered treatment either voluntarily or compulsorily. These studies tend to focus on criminal issues such as rates of recidivism or on psychological profiling of offenders. Because of the samples used, they miss the experiences of those who are sexually attracted but do not act on their attraction. They are also likely to miss the experiences of those who, whether they act on their attraction or not, reject any notion that they are 'sick' and should seek any kind of voluntary 'treatment'. Thus forensic samples will only be able to access that small proportion of paedophiles who (1) commit sexual offences against children and (2) are apprehended and (3) are prosecuted and (4) are convicted and (5) are approached to take part in a study and (6) agree to participate. Similarly, psychiatric studies will only be able to access samples who have either voluntarily agreed to enter therapy, or have been compelled to take part in some form of treatment as part of their rehabilitation, and are invited to participate in a study and agree to participate. These studies often rule out those who are only incarcerated for a short time, as it usually takes a number of months to set up a project, negotiate access, set up interviews and complete them, all of which requires a fairly stable population. Therefore, again, sudies generally end up conducting research only on the worst offenders, who will have received the longest prison sentences and are therefore relatively accessible to researchers. People who receive shorter prison sentences are also less likely to be offered treatment either inside prison or once they are released on probation – therefore again making it likely that research will only be carried out on more serious offenders.

Of those paedophiles who do not offend (or are not caught), an unknown proportion may define themselves as having a psychiatric or psychological problem and therefore consider voluntary psychiatric treatment, therapy or counselling. Of this unknown proportion, it is likely that a number who consider treatment will not in fact ever enter treatment because they will be too apprehensive of the potential legal and social consequences to come forward and identify themselves even to a member of the helping professions. Of those who do, and discuss their sexual attraction to children openly with the professional, it is again relatively unlikely that they will be engaged in any form of research. The consequences of all these constraints on researching people sexually attracted to children means that samples, however derived, will tend to be skewed in one direction or another. Those who remain outside the scrutiny of most research projects are known by some researchers as being in the 'dunkelfeld' (or 'dark field', that is, at large in the community and unknown to the authorities): one recent German study, at the Institute of Sexology and Sexual Medicine at the Freie und Humboldt-Universität in Berlin encouraged paedophiles in the 'dark field' to come forward for research as part of free confidential counselling (Beier 2004). However, the Berlin study has been the only one so far using such a methodology and again its focus is not on the everyday life experiences of the paedophile but predominantly on psychological attributes.

Alongside these forensic and clinical studies there have been a small number of more 'alternative' projects arising from a more or less explicitly apologist stance. These studies are generally, from the evidence available, conducted by men who identify themselves or who are linked to some degree with the 'pederast' or 'boy-lover' movement (although this is not always the position which is taken publicly). Broadly academic published studies on paedophiles who are not incarcerated or undergoing therapy but are living at large in the community have included those conducted by Parker Rossman (1976), Glenn Wilson and David Cox (1983), Edward Brongersma (1986), Theo Sandfort (1987) and Chin-Keung Li *et al.* (1990), with various more recent non-academic studies by David Riegel (for example, see Riegel 2007), and a doctoral study by Richard Yuill, awarded by Glasgow University in 2005, which is not yet in the public domain. Of these authors, it is perhaps Li who, in his writing, seems to stand back the furthest from his subject matter and interrogates his findings from the broadest perspective. (A fuller discussion of these and other texts on 'boy-lovers' or 'child-lovers' is presented in Goode, forthcoming.)

Other than using forensic or clinical samples often drawn from prison populations or relying on the reports presented by those more or less sympathetic to the pro-paedophile movement, how is it possible to find out more about this deeply hidden and stigmatised group of people? The straightforward initial answer is of course that we must ask them. Only self-defined paedophiles themselves can begin to tell us what it is like to experience sexual attraction to children and how they feel about having such a sexual attraction. Nevertheless, like any data, information from paedophiles – as from any source – must not be taken directly on its own terms but be critically and rigorously analysed. This current research project started from a different position from either the 'mainstream', often psychology-based, perspective or the 'alternative' apologist perspective and the data for this study – obtained through questionnaire-responses, interviews and more informal communications – have been analysed using a perspective which critiques traditional masculine attitudes to sex and sexuality.

This chapter is comprised of three sections. Section I provides a brief overview of how the MAA Daily Lives Research Project came about. This was a difficult project to set up for various reasons and Section II outlines some of the background factors which affected the climate within which this research was planned, while Section III summarises the major ethical and methodological difficulties encountered during the planning and conduct of the research. The next chapter then looks at how the project was conducted, and the following chapters provide details of the findings.

Section I: The origins of the MAA Daily Lives Research Project

My research began originally with a leaflet which I found inside a magazine. The magazine was one aimed at middle-class professionals, and the leaflet was produced by a well-known national charity. The leaflet was about paedophiles. The cover of the leaflet was designed to look like torn-out newspapers headlines and contained statements such as 'Britain's worst paedophile' and 'Paedophile groomed boy, 14, for sex ring'. The leaflet claimed, 'Because paedophiles are organised, we must be better organised. Because they are cunning, we must be more intelligent. Because they are many, we must have the support of many more…the more of them there are, the more we need you.' The depiction of child sexual abusers which it presented was that they were radically different from other people: cunning, devious, manipulative, frightening, a growing threat, without humanity, evil.

This leaflet worried me. It did not ring true. What many studies and theories over the past century or so have repeatedly shown is that people are not monsters. There is no 'us' and 'them'. No one is intrinsically and whole-heartedly evil, just as no one is able to be whole-heartedly good. We are all capable of inflicting terrible pain and cruelty, and we are all capable of selfless and compassionate caring. A simplistic vision of 'paedophiles' as 'others', different from us, did not reflect the nuanced reality studied by social scientists. It also did not reflect the experiences of those women and men who have spoken out about their experiences of childhood sexual abuse, often committed by people they loved and trusted – not by monsters they feared and hated. Perhaps most importantly, it did not allow for the basic fact about sexual abuse: that it affects around a quarter of all girls and at least a tenth of all boys (Itzin 2006). It makes much more sense to see that there is no clear distinction between 'us' and 'them' – as discussed in Chapter 1 adult sexual attraction to children, and adult sexual contact with children, affects a very large percentage of our population. My response to the 'paedophile' leaflet led me on to conduct a thought experiment, which ultimately resulted in my research and hence this book.

Imagine for a moment that you are an adult (or adolescent) of reasonable intelligence, typical morals, and good standing in the community. You have found yourself over the last few months or years increasingly worried by your sexual feelings towards children. You feel that you could really use some information, advice and support to help you deal with this very disturbing situation. What do you do?

Do you:

1. Discuss your experiences with your spouse/partner or other nearest and dearest?
2. Seek the advice of a professional – perhaps your local medical doctor or social worker?
3. Trot down to your library and see if you can borrow a book on 'Self Help for Paedophiles' or similar?
4. Quietly go online when no one's looking and see what you can find out there?

The most likely option for many people is to choose the relative anonymity of the Internet for their first foray into self-discovery. Their first step will be to type a word, for example 'paedophile' or 'pedophile', into a search engine such as Google. Google results are page-ranked according to an algorithm which provides the most relevant and commonly accessed web-pages first. Often within four clicks or less (depending on levels of online activism), an individual can enter an entirely legal pro-paedophile site (such as the Puellula site mentioned in the previous chapter, now defunct) where they can encounter a range of information, advice and support, including assurances that sexual attraction to children can be a highly positive experience, rewarding for both the adult and the child. It is these sites, the information they draw on, and the views and experiences of the people involved in them, which primarily formed the subject of my research. These are the alternative discourses around paedophilia and adult-child sexual contact which are so easily available online and yet which are so extraordinarily divergent from the everyday dominant mainstream discourses, whether those draw on the dry and stodgily unimaginative bureaucracy of social work practice or the – equally unhelpful – breathlessly sensationalist simplifications of the popular media.

Having been troubled by the concepts of 'the paedophile' which were implicit in the leaflet from the charity, I wrote two papers on 'rethinking paedophiles' which were presented at the British Sociological Association Medical Sociology Conference, York University, England, in 2005 and at the Interdisciplinary Conference on Wickedness and Human Evil, Salzburg, Austria, in 2006. In February 2006, I received a brief email from someone in the USA who had noticed an abstract of my paper published on the conference website and who requested a copy of my full paper. The email address suggested to me that the correspondent had emailed from a pro-paedophile website. I emailed back, offering a copy of my paper and tentatively indicating that I would be happy to correspond with people who self-identified as paedophile. The correspondent, 'Darren', replied:

> *Thank you for your response to my inquiry. … I experience the apparently congenital condition described as 'sexual attraction to children'. … I believe that there is a significant risk of harm to children who are involved in sexual relationships with adults, and do not support changing age of consent types of laws. I believe that child pornography is harmful to my community, as well as to the public at large. I believe that the repression this community of people live under forces our public efforts to extreme political views. … Outside of the issue of orientation, I am indistinguishable from larger society. I am conservative, Christian, and Republican; I voted for George Bush and support Tony Blair. … I am married and [a parent]. … I would be more than happy to engage in any dialogue that is useful to your work. I am human, and many times others do not realise that I share the same concerns and ambitions as they in society. I appreciate the work you are doing.*
>
> (Darren, personal communication 2006)

In later emails, Darren told me about having been 'beaten, stabbed, and sexually assaulted' over his orientation and referred to his belief that he would be killed because of people's knowledge of his paedophilia. Like David, whom we met in Chapter 1, Darren too became concerned about his orientation while he was still a young teenager at school. As someone who had himself been sexually abused as a child, Darren 'hated keeping secrets' so, unlike David, he made the decision that he must talk to someone about his feelings and told a school counsellor. Having told the counsellor, he was left to wait in her office for two anxious hours until she returned with a social worker who arranged for him to be admitted immediately to an adolescent psychiatric unit. On the way to the unit, the social worker made it clear to Darren how much she hated paedophiles. Within hours of first admitting to his worries, the terrified teenager found himself strapped spreadeagled to a bed with leather restraints while four adults stood around his bed. One adult unzipped Darren's trousers and held his penis in a pair of scissors, threatening to cut it off. Darren was convinced this was really going to happen. Since Darren was himself still only a child when this happened, this was certainly a strange form of 'child protection'. Darren pleaded to be allowed to see his parents and to get legal help. He was told that 'it was the judge who had ordered this treatment, and that no one would listen to him'. Darren's treatment involved being 'compelled to sit on a hard wood chair against a wall, for a period of seven days, from seven A.M. to eleven P.M. each day, with five minute breaks every two hours to use the bathroom under supervision, under coercion of restraint' if he refused to comply. Darren was 'subject to repeated restraining, for periods from twenty-four hours, to forty hours, over the next several years'. The treatment that Darren received at that time and subsequently did not 'cure' his paedophilia and did not encourage him to be open about his feelings or his activities. As he summed it up, 'I am numb to pain. This has been a difficult life, one I would not wish on anyone.' Like a suspect taken to Guantanamo Bay accused only of having socially unacceptable thoughts and beliefs, Darren was denied the due process of law and punished not for a criminal offence but for the potential harm which might be caused by his deviant thoughts. Rather than frightening him out of his paedophilic tendencies, however, the harsh treatment Darren received had the effect of radicalising him into vigorous political activism.

As well as telling me about his own experiences and views, Darren told me, 'I have met several hundred non-offending minor-attracted individuals. Many have told me that I am the first, and the last, person they will ever tell; it was not a risk they would take readily again but reached out to me in desperation.'

The fact that Darren was very active in the 'paedophile community' and that he had many contacts among self-defined 'minor-attracted adults' made him an ideal gatekeeper into this population. Given this fortuitous opening, I began to set up a project to collect data.

Section II: The background research climate

Having navigated my way through the intricacies of interviewing heroin-dependent mothers for my doctoral research, I naively assumed that researching MAAs would be fairly straightforward. Since the focus of my proposed research was not on criminal behaviour but on cultural issues of identity formation and on the fascinating and hitherto unresearched phenomenon of 'non-contact' paedophiles – those who are sexually attracted to children but choose not to act on that attraction – I believed that it was self-evident that my research would assist in child protection and also that it would help move us away from an hysterical and misguided obsession with evil child molesters. Events were to prove me quite wrong.

The study focused on the relatively new phenomenon of computer-mediated identity formation, as part of the wider and more traditional exploration of the negotiation of individual identity within communities.

There were four main research questions:

1. What are the discourses mediating the construction and negotiation of online identities among adults sexually attracted to children?
2. What information, advice and support is provided to its members by the online 'paedophile community'?
3. What are the key issues currently being debated within the online 'paedophile community'?
4. What are the implications of the research-findings for improving the level of child protection?

The research objectives were:

1. To locate and analyse legal textual material on the Internet: this includes pro- and anti-paedophile websites, news items, blogs, commentaries and discussion boards and podcasts, found through sites including Wikipedia, BBC Online, online newspapers and other sources. From the analysis of online material, to identify research themes and also to identify key activists in this area as potential research participants.
2. To make contact with key activists and other adults who self-define as sexually attracted to minors under the age of sixteen years and to invite them to participate in voluntary and confidential qualitative research which does not solicit information on illegal activities.
3. To request activists and others to act as key informants and gatekeepers into the community, and where entry is permitted to encourage the use of snowballing as a peer-recruitment method to contact further samples of MAAs.
4. From the samples available, to investigate questions relating to the social construction of a hidden and stigmatised community, and the construction, negotiation and management of identity.

As can be seen, there was no research focus on criminal behaviour or on child pornography. Nevertheless, to do this relatively uncontroversial and straight-forward piece of academic research I had to battle with over a year of suspicion and hostility, from early 2006 to mid-2007. Two larger, unrelated, processes were taking place at the time I began the research which ensured that it would not be plain sailing.

The first process was outside academic life and mainly located in the USA. Anti-paedophile online activists, and particularly Perverted Justice, began a campaign from 2003 onwards of actively working to have pro-paedophile websites closed down and individuals identified, 'outed' and if possible prosecuted. This campaign had some notable successes and between 2006 and 2008 the tenor of the pro-paedophile web-presence changed. Individuals who had previously felt relatively relaxed about posting messages and communicating with others now became far more suspicious and wary. I was frequently told that if I had conducted this research in 2006 I would have received considerably more responses than I could in 2007 or 2008. At the start of the research the 'participant coordinators group' were fully confident that I would receive around 200 responses. In the event I received fewer than sixty. Having the research delayed by ethics committees and bureaucratic considerations had damaged it irreparably. (I would like to note here that, although the work of Perverted Justice incidentally happened to reduce my access to a large sample from the online paedophile community, my comments on this volunteer organisation, here and elsewhere in this book, should not be taken as criticism. Perverted Justice does not make a clear distinction between those adults who are sexually attracted to children and those adults who intend to have sexual contact with children, nor does it make any distinction between those individuals or websites promoting sexual contact with children and those maintaining a law-abiding stance. This is very regrettable, but when Perverted Justice identifies and prevents men sexually abusing children, then any individual concerned about children can only approve. Since its inception, Perverted Justice has played a significant role in obtaining convictions against over 300 men who had actively sought sexual contact with children. They have done this by posing as children aged twelve to fifteen years old in chat rooms, responding when contacted by an adult man seeking sex and setting up meetings in a house. The man is arrested when he arrives at the house in order to have sex with a minor. In some cases, the details are truly chilling: in one case a man, expecting to have sex with a fourteen-year-old boy, brought his own five-year-old son along with him; other men bring guns; one man, Benjamin Brown, who had previously been convicted of raping a young girl, arrived to meet the decoy, 'Cami', with a rope, gags, handcuffs and a knife. In such cases one can only be profoundly grateful for the work of Perverted Justice.)

The second process affecting the research came into play in the academic community within the UK from the early 2000s onwards and involved an increase in managerialism and bureaucratisation. This led to a climate of caution in taking on any research which could possibly be regarded as potentially harmful in any way. After scandals such as the disproportionate number of deaths of infant cardiac-surgery patients at Bristol Royal Infirmary in the late 1990s, strong bureaucratic processes of ethics scrutiny were set up across all UK research institutions (for example see Economic and Social Research Council 2005), modelled on the specific traditions of ethics review committees required in medical research and less sympathetic to the more fluid and nuanced practices of social science. As society itself has arguably become generally more risk-aware and risk-averse (Giddens 2002; Mythen

2004), it has been said that the movement set in motion by the risk society can be summarised simply in the statement 'I am afraid!' (Beck 1992: 49). However, not all risk is taken equally seriously: risk governance experts remind us that acceptable risk levels vary 'by orders of magnitude among different policy domains' (Hood *et al.* 2004: 171), and indeed some risks may be overestimated while other serious threats are ignored.

With the rise of managerialism, research governance mechanisms, risk assessment and auditing of paper trails have become the watchwords of academic research. This increasingly timorous risk-averse climate has arguably deprofessionalised academic practice, reducing academic freedom and autonomy. A campaign, Academics for Academic Freedom, has been set up to counter this trend, but has made little headway. All research regarded as involving 'sensitive topics' (including all research on sexual issues) has become wellnigh excluded from universities, due in part to the negative consequences for the academics concerned (Goode 2007a; Sikes 2008). Research on such areas is too often left only to journalists but they, too, have their own difficulties to contend with and, in a sound-bite culture, careful and courageous in-depth investigation of social topics such as paedophilia has too often been replaced by a tendency to oversimplify (Franklin and Parton 1991; Thompson 1998); a tendency exacerbated by a moral and intellectual climate which stigmatises and scapegoats rather than analyses and reflects (Silverman and Wilson 2002; Kitzinger 2004; Richards 2007).

These two larger-scale factors of increased online anti-paedophile activism and reduced academic freedom affected – and damaged – the research, but another process was also taking place. This process was closer to home and seemed to revolve around the issue of legitimacy, whether personal, academic or methodological.

The first aspect of legitimacy was along the lines of, 'What kind of person would want to research paedophiles?' Being made to think about paedophilia arouses uncomfortable feelings, so (as with tabloid newspaper articles) the discomfort is resolved in the identification of a scapegoat. The person responsible for arousing such feelings is made a scapegoat and that person is then rejected so that they alone carry the unpleasant feelings which otherwise the group would have to own and address. Doubts were cast on me as an individual, and on my motivation for wanting to be associated with this topic and wanting to immerse myself in this murky world. In psychoanalytic terms, this was also a form of projection. One way to reduce the felt anxiety arising from thinking about paedophiles and the sexual abuse of children is to project those difficult feelings outwards, for example by pushing them onto the researcher, and then to push them further away by rejecting the researcher and undermining or delaying the successful progress of the research.

The second aspect of legitimacy was, 'What discipline ought properly to research paedophiles?' Again, this tended to be a distancing mechanism but more basically it betrayed a view that some disciplines (social work, criminology, forensic psychiatry) are trustworthy and can legitimately research serious topics such as child sexual abuse while other disciplines (cultural studies, sociology) are untrustworthy, naïve, frivolous and irrelevant. This fight over disciplines (and it was a fight) seemed to be embedded in a distrust of any research which is purely academic, which seeks to explore culture and develop theory, rather than research which is conducted by practitioners and is strictly practice-based, applied research, with little critique of underlying worldviews. Ultimately, this questioning of legitimacy suggested a basic distrust of the value of pure academic research and perhaps academia itself, which – in the context of higher education – was very disheartening.

The third question provoked by my wish to do this research was, 'How should such research be done?' Curiously, colleagues seem to prefer that this research on paedophiles should ideally be conducted without ever having to enter into the presence of any paedophile, or be in any way contaminated by any contact with any paedophile. This is an interesting position to hold. Paedophiles – that is, adults who find themselves sexually attracted to children and youth aged under sixteen years – are so demonised in contemporary society *whether or not they act on that sexual attraction* that I was told that I was not allowed to interview them in my office because I must not facilitate their presence on campus. An email from senior management implied that I was expected to complete a formal risk assessment for every interview conducted and also informed me that: 'You are aware that you must not interview or otherwise facilitate the presence of any paedophiles, self declared or otherwise, on University property' (personal communication, June 2007). The fact that, in a population of around 500 staff and over 5,000 students, there was likely already to be at least one or two paedophiles 'self-declared or otherwise' on university property did not apparently affect this argument, even when I pointed it out. Such is the force of a moral panic.

I also must not go to locations overseas where I might be able to meet with and interview any paedophiles (including rather eminent, distinguished and scholarly old professors) just in case they corrupted or attacked me. When individual people become so corrosively vilified, not because of what they *do* but because of what they *are,* it is certainly time that sociologists and other students of culture study this phenomenon. As an example of the moral panic induced by the mere thought of paedophiles, I was solemnly informed by a senior campus official that there was a problem with 'paedophiles' crouching outside the windows of student accommodation and spying on female students. Given that students are aged at least eighteen years old, this conflation of 'paedophile' with 'sex offender' was both significant and absurd. The concept of 'paedophile' was also conflated with the concept of 'violent sex offender' and I was warned that, if I met any paedophiles, I must make sure I had a personal alarm with me at all times, in case of attack. The likelihood, as a middle-aged adult, of my being sexually attacked by a paedophile seems remote. The injunction against interviewing paedophiles on campus in fact exposed me, if anything, to a greater level of risk. Because I could not interview them securely in my office, with colleagues in adjoining rooms who could have rescued me if needed, I had to meet unknown men in locations including their homes. The only time I felt even mildly apprehensive was sitting in a room in an otherwise empty house with a rather excitable interviewee standing between myself and the door.

Having outlined some of the wider context within which I struggled even to begin the research, I will now briefly consider some of the ethical and methodological problems thrown up by the details of the project itself.

Section III: Ethical and methodological challenges of the project

Before commencing a discussion of the ethical and methodological issues raised by this research, it is relevant to make a point about the epistemological base on which the project is grounded. I seem to be different from many other researchers in this field in my understanding of what constitutes knowledge. It is noticeable that most of those researching and writing on paedophilia – whether psychologists, sexologists or biologists – come from an academic tradition which espouses a view of scientific knowledge as having the capacity – and the goal – of being objective, neutral, value-free, able to make universal claims and seeking towards a single, unifying truth which can be captured and tested by replicable experiments on identifiable and measurable variables. This approach is summed up, for example, in the claim by Jones (1991: 289):

> As in all research, the study of intimate intergenerational relationships, pedophilia, child sexuality and related issues will be effective only to the extent that professionals involved in such study resolve to identify and reject emotionality in all its forms and influences. Terminology must be neutral and each researcher and author must acknowledge the probability that society's emotional reactions are affecting her or his results or interpretations.

This is a typical plea for what is regarded as the desirable and attainable goal of unemotional neutrality, and what is also typical here is that Jones, in the article in which he argues this, is himself presenting an emotional plea for greater sympathy (for adult male paedophiles). When discussing human phenomena we all, as researchers, have to acknowledge our own humanity and our own lived reality – our gendered, sexed body and our autobiographical histories. No matter how much we might try, we cannot come to a study of people's experiences without bringing our own experiences with us, either as prejudices and biases or potentially as resources, used consciously and intentionally. Each one of us, when we think of 'intimate intergenerational relationships, pedophilia, child sexuality and related issues' as Jones terms it, remembers and reflects on our own experiences and those of people we know. Based on our epistemological position, we can either attempt to reject this knowledge (which will still influence us unconsciously if not otherwise) or we can accept the inevitable and make use of our lived and 'situated' knowledge to inform and deepen our understanding (Haraway 1988). We fit what we learn into our existing schema and thereby develop them. As social scientists we aim to do this transparently and reflexively, using our own experiences to sensitise us. The social scientist, working in this tradition, becomes the research tool, bringing insights as well as inevitable blind spots to the research. This avoids the 'fallacy of value-neutrality' (Kohlberg 1981) and the fiction of the 'objective' and dispassionate scientist, observing and judging the world from some privileged, god-like position (Haraway 1988; Harding 1991). There is no universal, objective point from which to observe, and certainly not when it comes to something as emotionally charged as children and sexuality. This epistemological position was the background and starting point for my enquiry into understanding adult sexual attraction to children, and it informed my ethical stance throughout the research process.

The main ethical consideration which concerned me throughout the project was the possibility of potential harm to respondents, as there was a risk of accidental disclosure consequent on their research participation. This was minimised first through informed consent, which detailed how the project was being carried out so that respondents could choose their level of risk (for example, through the email account they chose to contact me through), and second through immediately breaking links between data and identifiable individuals as soon as data was collected, and maintaining the anonymity and confidentiality of all material. The only exception to this confidentiality rule occurred when previously unreported criminal activity was disclosed to me and the respondent was identifiable. In this one case, as the Information Sheet had made clear throughout, the information was passed on directly to the police when it became clear that a child might be at immediate risk of significant harm.

From the beginning, the intention of this project was that my approach to the respondents would be fully consonant with my own ethical and epistemological framework and with my professional practice as described in the British Sociological Association's *Statement of Ethical Practice* (2002: para. 14) which states, 'research relationships should be characterised, whenever possible, by trust and integrity'. This maxim was followed and all my research was conducted as openly as possible. It would have been possible, for example, to conduct aspects of this research covertly, for example by 'lurking' on discussion boards. Journalists and some researchers have indeed collected data on the online paedophile community by 'lurking' on public-access chat-sites and monitoring the comments made (for example, see Eichenwald 2006). I deliberately chose not to use this procedure, partly because I felt uncomfortable with the ethical implications of 'lurking' and also because I wished to avoid the practical implications of attempting to quote comments without identifying writers. I have used this method only where such quotations are already clearly in the public domain (such as published on Wikipedia or already quoted on other sites such as Wikisposure). I made the decision to rely instead on what respondents chose quite consciously and deliberately to write or say to me in a context in which they knew I was conducting research. Similarly, I could have chosen to present myself as being sexually attracted to children (which some respondents appeared to assume in any case), but I did not. I worked hard to be as open and transparent as possible with all participants, even where this may have compromised the quality of the data obtained because of objections on the part of respondents to my acknowledged worldview, which I occasionally could not avoid disclosing. At the same time, I worked hard to build rapport with the community and to treat all respondents with the respect and consideration which would be accorded any other individual. Again, this conforms to the BSA *Statement of Ethical Practice* (2002: para. 10) that 'Sociologists, when they carry out research, enter into personal and moral relationships with those they study': this moral relationship must include respect which in turn includes showing respect for certain views. For example, the Information Sheet (see Appendix B) used neutral language which echoed the terminology used by members of the community; this is a reason the term 'minor-attracted adult' was used in preference to 'paedophile'. The *Statement* (BSA 2002: para. 11) comments that the goal of research does not provide 'an entitlement to override the rights of others' and this project accepted that the 'rights of others' includes the right to their own opinions (although not the right to undertake criminal activity). This approach to language choice and other sensitivities reflects my epistemological stance as someone who is concerned with the 'situated knowledges' (Haraway 1988) of respondents and it also fits with the *Statement* which comments that:

> Sociologists have a responsibility to ensure that the physical, social and psychological well-being of research participants is not adversely affected by the research. They should strive to protect the rights of those they study, their interests, sensitivities and privacy, while recognising the difficulty of balancing potentially conflicting interests.
>
> (BSA 2002: para. 13)

I had previously experienced and analysed aspects of conducting 'sensitive' research in relation to my work on researching substance-dependent mothers (Goode 2000; Goode 2007b). This had included the dilemmas of researching and building rapport with a hidden and stigmatised population and the development of research relationships with respondents, including the ethical issue of providing (and withholding) personal information as part of actively negotiating respectful relationships within a democratic research paradigm.

The use of the Internet as a primary means of collecting data is a difficult and emerging field of debate in research ethics. The *Statement of Ethical Practice* states:

> Members should take special care when carrying out research via the Internet. Ethical standards for internet research are not well developed as yet. Eliciting informed consent, negotiating access agreements, assessing the boundaries between the public and the private, and ensuring the security of data transmissions are all problematic in internet research. Members

who carry out research online should ensure that they are familiar with ongoing debates on the ethics of internet research, and might wish to consider erring on the side of caution in making judgements affecting the well-being of online research participants.

(BSA 2002: para. 41)

An article on 'Ethical Issues in Qualitative Research on Internet Communities' (Eysenbach and Till 2001) divides Internet-based research into three types: passive analysis (such as analysis of website content); active analysis (where researchers participate in communications, for example on discussion boards); and 'traditional' analysis (where researchers identify themselves as such and gather online information using traditional methods). In these terms it could be said that the methodology of this project was to use passive analysis and traditional research. Passive analysis involves locating legal websites (including email discussion boards, blogs and podcasts), and using standard methods of textual analysis to analyse the material. Although such material was clearly all in the public domain (no subscription-only sites were accessed), there could have been legitimate resentment if postings or other 'conversations' had been subsequently analysed for research purposes: I have therefore not made use of such semi-public material. Eysenbach and Till state that 'On the Internet the dichotomy of private and public sometimes may not be appropriate, and communities may lie in between' (2001: 1104). They note, for example, that where quotations are taken from newsgroups or other mailing lists, it can be possible to link direct quotes back to an individual's email address, even where the researcher has removed this in the published research, if the quote is searched for using a sufficiently powerful search engine. I have therefore tried to treat all such material, including quotations, judiciously. Staying with Eysenbach and Till's typology, for the 'traditional' aspects of methodology, negotiating access agreement was done through gatekeepers who were able to discuss the research project with members of the online community and who were also in a position to recommend or advise against participation among potential respondents. Respondents subsequently made up their own minds on whether to contact the researcher or not, and what level of information to disclose. Data transmissions were done through a password-protected email account at my university and thus were as safe as any other email correspondence, while the email addresses used by those who contacted me tended to be generated from websites with a very high degree of security and untraceability.

Other than the unusually high level of potential harm to respondents, and the ethics peculiar to online research, this was a very ordinary social science research project. The overall research methodology was broadly similar to that used in my doctoral research, which had been reviewed and authorised by my local Regional Health Authority Ethics Committee. Standard methodologies of data collection were used, incorporating a grounded-theory approach (Glaser 1978; Glaser and Strauss 1967; Strauss 1987; Strauss and Corbin 1990;

Strauss and Corbin 1997) as ongoing data analysis suggested new research topics to explore and enabled the generation of new questions throughout the duration of the project. Thus the research focus of the study was repeatedly refined as material was collected. No questions were asked on individual identity or on criminal activity. Respondents (unless they chose to volunteer details) were both anonymous and (legally and pragmatically) untraceable. I had no control over who chose to participate, although the Information Sheet (see Appendix B) explained who I was looking for. Since respondents were anonymous, it was impossible to verify the identity of any respondent, so all the data, including the information on age, gender, sexual orientation and so on had to be taken on trust. Although this potentially means that non-suitable respondents could have given data which has subsequently been included in the analysis, it is unlikely that anyone who is not a self-defined paedophile would have wished to have been included or indeed would have been included, particularly since the gatekeepers are very much attuned to the issue of infiltration by vigilantes, journalists and others. In fact, a concern over age meant that some willing participants were at first excluded (and got quite annoyed about it). In order to be scrupulous about informed consent and to avoid including minors (in any jurisdiction), it was necessary to define participants as only those aged over twenty-one years. When potential respondents younger than twenty-one contacted me and asked to participate, which happened on several occasions, I explained the reason why not. Individuals younger than twenty-one years did, however, wish to participate and at first gatekeepers prevented them. This issue was then resolved by allowing those aged under twenty-one to participate, but keeping their details separate. (This is discussed further in the following chapter.) What is significant here is that the respondents, and the gatekeepers, did not attempt to 'get around' what they perceived as an irritating barrier by choosing simply to lie to me: instead, they followed the rules but objected openly to them and we found a way of resolving the issue while maintaining the integrity of the project.

Once the data were received, it was essential to guard responses carefully. The BSA *Statement of Ethical Practice* (2002: para. 36) states that:

> Appropriate measures should be taken to store research data in a secure manner. Members should have regard to their obligations under the Data Protection Acts. Where appropriate and practicable, methods for preserving anonymity should be used including the removal of identifiers, the use of pseudonyms and other technical means for breaking the link between data and identifiable individuals.

In conformity with the provisions of the UK Data Protection Act 1995 and the guidelines of the BSA, all the data collected had identifiers removed and replaced by pseudonyms to break the link between data and identifiable individuals. Data were stored either as anonymised extracts within files on a password-protected computer or as complete anonymised printouts kept securely. Because transcripts were kept only as hard-copy print-outs for security reasons, and free-text rather than pre-coded answers had been asked for, this meant that manual rather than computer-assisted analysis was the main method used. Working closely with the transcripts helped me to think about possible connections and themes, but the disadvantage was that multi-variate analysis was impossible to carry out.

Accidental disclosure of confidential material was not the only risk to be avoided. As noted earlier, there was a pervasive sense among some colleagues that – since the term 'paedophile' is felt to be subsumed by the term 'violent sex offender' – I put myself at risk even by meeting paedophiles. The BSA *Statement of Ethical Practice* (2002: para. 8) states that: 'Social researchers face a range of potential risks to their safety. Safety issues need to be con-sidered in the design and conduct of social research projects and procedures should be adopted to reduce the risk to researchers.' The main concern for me was staying on the right side of the law. I obtained legal advice from two lawyers (one in the UK and one in the USA) and followed the advice given by my local police authority on avoiding illegal websites and ensuring that no illegal material was downloaded. A very senior local police officer with responsibility for overseeing public protection in this field was particularly helpful in reading through draft questionnaires and advising on wording: he also checked my online statement, posted on the research website.

Wider issues included the well-being not just of the respondents and myself, but also my institution and wider stakeholders. The BSA *Statement of Ethical Practice* (2002: para. 6) states that: 'Members have responsibility both to safeguard the proper interests of those involved in or affected by their work, and to report their findings accurately and truthfully.' The 'proper interests' of all stakeholders in this subject, including the interests of children, and my endeavour to report findings accurately and truthfully are, I hope, fully reflected in the content of this book.

While this project was being negotiated, an issue which gave particular con-cern to ethics committees was that of informed consent and therefore it is worth spending a little time exploring this. The *Statement of Ethical Practice* states that:

> As far as possible participation in sociological research should be based on the freely given informed consent of those studied. This implies responsibility on the sociologist to explain in appropriate detail, and in terms meaningful to participants, what the research is about, who is undertaking and financing it, why it is being undertaken, and how it is to be disseminated and used.
>
> (BSA 2002: para. 16)

The *Statement* also says:

> In some situations access to a research setting is gained via a 'gatekeeper'. In these situations members should adhere to the principle of obtaining

informed consent directly from the research participants to whom access is required, while at the same time taking account of the gatekeepers' interest.

(BSA 2002: para. 25)

In many ways, this was a very straightforward issue. Respondents gave their consent to the research by choosing to participate in it. They were free to refuse to participate or to terminate their participation at any time. Although I was initially dependent entirely on gatekeepers to advertise the research, circulate information and invite volunteers, once contact with a participant was made, I could then aim to establish a research relationship directly with that participant rather than by way of the gatekeeper. There was no possibility of respondents taking part in this research without their consent as respondents voluntarily chose to make the initial and any subsequent contact. I was quite unable to make contact with any participants who had not disclosed their email address or other contact method. When a respondent contacted me and provided a method for replying, I would check with them that they had received the Information Sheet and had the opportunity to provide evidence of informed consent.

One request that the ethics committee made initially was that all respondents provide hand-signed forms to indicate informed consent. It did not appear obvious to the committee that individuals with profoundly stigmatised identities, answering an anonymous online questionnaire, would not appreciate being asked to print out and sign a form, which would then presumably also need to be sent by mail (including airmail) back to me. I explained that it was likely that respondents would refrain from signing consent forms or in any other way revealing their identity. This included pseudonyms or 'nicks' already chosen by the respondents. Any email addresses or Internet nicknames used by the respondents are regarded as evidence of their identity, and so are subject to the same level of anonymity and confidentiality as 'real' names, the only exception being where such nicknames are used to show authorship of published material, for example in Wikipedia entries or as web-editors.

The question of insisting on potential research participants providing signed evidence of their informed consent to participate has been discussed in a number of research articles, notably in 'Signing Your Life Away? Why Research Ethics Committees (REC) Shouldn't Always Require Written Confirmation that Participants in Research Have Been Informed of the Aims of a Study and Their Rights – The Case of Criminal Populations', a commentary in the peer-reviewed journal *Sociological Research Online* (Coomber 2002). Coomber makes the point that research ethics committees have tended to adopt uncritically the extant model of research ethics rooted in a medical model of invasive procedures such as surgical or drugs trials. This medical model is at odds with the ethical requirements of social science, particularly when researching hidden or criminal populations. Coomber (2002: para 1.3) states 'Asking participants to sign a form admitting to illegal acts therefore actually contradicts other aspects of most REC criteria rendering them, in certain circumstances, inconsistent and inappropriate.' It also lays the research participants and researcher open to greater levels of risk as any research material on criminal activity is then more likely to be used as evidence in criminal proceedings. Coomber discusses a number of situations where participants end up signing 'Mickey Mouse' or other pseudonyms on the consent forms, thereby creating a situation where rules are followed meaninglessly and researchers are forced to 'play a game' with the research ethics committees. Truman, in 'Ethics and the Ruling Relations of Research Production' (2003), makes a broader comment on the ways in which ethical and research governance can protect institutional interests, without necessarily providing an effective means to address the moral obligations and responsibilities of researchers. She highlights how RECs, operating within a traditional positivist research paradigm, frequently assume a role to 'protect' dependent and 'vulnerable' research 'subjects'. Such an approach may be not only inappropriate but also questionable in relation to participatory research methodology. As she points out, 'Researchers working within qualitative and/or participatory research paradigms are often acutely aware of ethical dilemmas contained within the process of conducting research with vulnerable groups, but try to address such dilemmas within an emergent process consistent with conducting democratic research' which she characterises as 'some of the most user-friendly approaches to social research' (Truman 2003: paragraph 1.1). These issues formed the basis for a national project, *Informed Consent and the Research Process,* and are developed further in an article in the *International Journal of Social Research Methodology* (Crow *et al.* 2006). This article, on 'Research Ethics and Data Quality, the Implications of Informed Consent', discusses how changing patterns of research governance are affecting the collection of research data. The authors suggest that there are problems associated with '*too much* attention' being paid to consent procedures which 'risks narrowing of research agendas if certain social groups or topics become unresearchable' (Crow *et al.* 2006: 95, emphases in original).

In this project, research respondents may or may not have been involved in criminal activity (which was of course not a focus of the research) and in many senses they were not a 'vulnerable' population, as they tended, on the evidence of the data given, to be highly educated, well informed, middle class and confident. They seemed to find the idea of signing a consent form to indicate their informed consent to the research both patronising and somewhat ludicrous. Rather than 'play the game', they simply politely ignored any such requests. Meanwhile, they ensured that they were in fact highly informed about the research, demonstrating this by (again, very politely) alluding to specific information about me, as discussed earlier. For example, one gatekeeper commented in an email, 'I read your brief bio on past occupations and found it very heartening', gently making the point that he had deliberately made the effort to find out about me. Thus, not only the project but also the researcher as an individual were being carefully 'checked out' as part of the decision-making process on whether to participate in the research. Such intensive scrutiny goes beyond traditional notions of 'informed consent' and implies a much more dynamic and 'democratic' process of participation, as Truman (2003) has suggested.

Having set out in this chapter some of the background and challenges encountered by attempting this research, the following chapter now recounts how the research was actually conducted and how members of the 'online paedophile community' responded to it.

4   Running the Minor-Attracted Adults Daily Lives Project

Introduction

Having provided some details on the setting up of the MAA Daily Lives Research Project in the previous chapter, this chapter now turns to look at what happened and how the project did eventually take place. This chapter is a sad tale of how a moral panic (Goode and Ben-Yehuda 1994; Critcher 2003) plays itself out in real life, with otherwise rational and sensible individuals caught up in a state of hysteria which appears to prevent the capacity to think clearly and independently (for other recent discussions on a similar theme, see Sikes 2008; Jenkins 2009). I hope that the following section will provide a reminder to those in the future of what the 'paedophile panic' looked like (and felt like) in 2006–7. As discussed in the previous chapter, my work in this area was not unique. For example, Richard Yuill had in 2005 successfully if controversially completed his doctoral study at Glasgow University in Scotland, supervised by David T. Evans, on 'age-discrepant' relationships between men and boys. Yuill was stoutly defended by his university who insisted on his academic freedom to research, but other researchers were less fortunate. In the UK, campaigns such as Academics for Academic Freedom (afaf.org.uk) set out clear statements and assist in providing a climate in which academic research can be conducted, but no one can campaign against those informal and subtle micro-processes of glances and unspoken words which create the most insidious undermining.

As a colleague of mine, working in a professional rather than an academic setting, discovered to his astonishment, just the suggestion of trying to understand paedophiles casts instant suspicion. During discussions on organising a conference on child protection, my colleague mooted the suggestion that, rather than the constant focus on victims, it might be useful to think about the perpetrators and try to understand their perspective. It took a mere twenty minutes or so of frozen hostility to realise he had said the wrong thing and to learn not to do that again. Perhaps I am less attuned to social cues, or perhaps I felt that this was too important an area of research to fall prey to those techniques of silencing. It probably helped in this research that I am a woman – but even that did not fully protect me from rumour.

In an academic environment the most damning rumour, and the hardest one to protect against, is that 'there are concerns' about the ethics of the research. This is like trying to pin down smoke. As I found, as soon as one nebulous 'concern' is identified and addressed, other 'concerns' emerge and waft obscurely through committee minutes, meeting rooms, social spaces – through the university and out into the wider world. 'There are concerns' is not something which can be adequately addressed by rigorous ethics scrutiny, as no one need actually articulate anything other than vague notions that there is 'risk' (to whom? Why?) or that there are 'issues'. Some of these 'concerns' are a covert expression of what could be termed 'tabloidophobia' – a horror that the more aggressively anti-intellectual of the tabloid newspapers could somehow come knocking and embarrass everyone. It certainly felt at the time as though my career and my reputation had been permanently damaged by choosing to research in this area. Shortly after I had published a brief article voicing my frustration (Goode 2007a), the process of ethics scrutiny was finally completed and by early summer 2007 I was at last able to begin the main data collection. In my experience, 'there are concerns' is ultimately not something which is amenable to open and robust debate where genuine questions over approaches or research methods can be clearly expressed and dealt with, and in the end this form of moral panic can be combated simply by standing firm and getting on with the job.

In this chapter, Section I outlines the process from first contact with Darren in February 2006 to beginning the main data collection in summer 2007. Data collection was finally completed by January 2008. During the many months of negotiating ethics approval, it was essential to maintain good working relations with the members of the paedophile community, and this is discussed in Section II, along with consideration of other aspects of working with this community.

Section I: How the research project was conducted

This section describes the process of contacting paedophiles and investigating their beliefs and experiences. Having established contact with Darren quite by chance, and discovering that he could put me in touch with 'hundreds' of paedophiles, almost all of whom were not known to the authorities but were living hidden lives in the community, I realised I had a unique opportunity. I continued to communicate with Darren and built rapport and trust. I needed to trust that Darren was not going to selectively choose which respondents I could access, or feed information to them, or set up a 'party line' on what to say which would distort the data I could receive. At the same time, Darren needed to trust that I would not attempt to 'out' any participants and that I would use the information entrusted to me respectfully.

My first priority was to design a research project to take advantage of this extraordinary opportunity. Together with other colleagues and with members of the paedophile community, I drafted and refined sets of questions to explore. At the same time, I wrote up an application for ethics approval from my university and a funding application to travel to the USA to run focus groups. Having begun the project in February 2006, the date for the focus groups was set for July 2006. Darren now set up an 'participant coordinators group' of around four key members of the paedophile community, to work with him on project-managing the logistics of bringing a large group of paedophiles together in one place for the focus-group interviews. (The 'participant coordinators group' doubtless also did its best to steer the research towards the best outcome for the paedophile community but, since this was predictable, it became simply another part of the data for me to research.) An activist, 'Paul Fisher', took on the logistics of the project and set up a website to advertise and coordinate the research, with a very professional-looking logo for what was now termed the MAA Daily Lives Project (see Appendix A for a copy of the logo). At the same time, I set up a university-based advisory group to assist me with the project, drawing on the expertise of academics and professionals involved in this field. This advisory group was under the aegis of the University of Winchester's Research and Policy Centre for the Study of Faith and Well-being in Communities, of which I was Director.

The first glitches in the process began when it was insisted, at the UK end, that I be accompanied on the research visit and, one by one, potential team members dropped out. A colleague was found to accompany me, but concerns apparently remained. The main concern (or possibly unconscious wish) appeared to be that I would be physically attacked by enraged or mentally unstable paedophiles, or beaten up by vigilantes, or arrested by the police for aiding and abetting criminal activities. There was also a fear that, by researching paedophiles and child sexual abuse, I would bring my institution into disrepute. The power of the tabloid or 'red-top' popular newspapers to shape public policy affected the decision-making of the institution. Perhaps people also felt that I would 'turn to the dark side' or that, merely by wanting to learn about paedophiles' experiences, I had already become a suspect outsider. The ethics approval process dragged on: concerns were raised, dealt with, and further concerns raised, in a seemingly endless cycle. Risk assessments were required. Review by external advisors was required. Further review by other external advisors was required. Police advice was required. Legal advice was required. Further legal advice was required. It was demanded that I provide paper copies of every email I had written or received in relation to the project (the only condition to which I objected and with which I did not comply). Further concerns were raised. The deadline for the focus groups loomed ever closer. When Paul Fisher informed me that respondents had taken leave from work and were now ready to book and pay for flights to attend the focus groups, I had to make a decision. After months of planning and preparation, with under six weeks to go to the actual interviews, I cancelled the visit as it was clear I could not guarantee that ethics sign-off would take place in time. The unique opportunity had been lost.

A back-up plan was developed, involving not face-to-face meetings but an online questionnaire which would be publicised on pro-paedophile websites and message boards. As with the proposed focus group research, the basic methodology of the revised project remained that of developing trust and a working relationship with key members who could operate as 'gatekeepers' for me into the international English-language online paedophile community. Through them, I could gain privileged entry into the online community and so carry out research on the views and experiences of self-defined paedophiles living at large in society. Further ethics scrutiny and funding applications were set up. Three different versions of the questionnaire were developed, piloted, refined and administered. Finally, as provisional and eventually full ethics approval were received, data began to come in and important findings began to emerge.

In addition to the online questionnaire, which had now become the main data collection tool for the project, I was able to meet with key individuals, including four self-identified paedophiles, for face-to-face conversations and recorded interviews. Only one of these was known to the authorities as a paedophile and, on the occasions when we met, he was in prison and therefore I was not allowed to take in pen or paper to make notes. With the other individuals, I arranged tape-recordings or written notes. In addition, I corresponded by telephone and email with a number of individuals. When individuals emailed me, I made sure that I stated (and repeated where necessary) that I was a researcher and therefore whatever they told me might be used as data. When they telephoned me, I made sure they realised if I was taking notes as they spoke. Alongside contacts with individuals known to be sympathetic to the pro-paedophile position, I met or corresponded with significant individuals from the academic, sexological, legal, criminal, probation, treatment and child protection fields, both nationally and internationally.

The Information Sheet and Questionnaire for participants are shown in Appendix B and C respectively. The Information Sheet was provided for anyone considering completing the questionnaire, to ensure that they understood what the research was about, who was conducting it, how the data would be treated, and the circumstances under which anonymity and confidentiality would *not* be assured. I provided this information in a separate document to the Questionnaire, to allow people to read it and consider the implications of responding before beginning to answer the questions. As discussed in the section on ethics, completing the Questionnaire was taken as indicating informed consent to participation in the project. The preface to the Questionnaire again drew attention to the Information Sheet, to ensure that it had been read and understood before the Questionnaire was completed. While I was developing this project, I was also conducting background research to consider the whole question of 'everyday paedophiles' more deeply (Goode, forthcoming), including an analysis of the British context (Goode 2008a, 2008b) and a comparison of the cinematic and Australian press constructions of paedophilia (Green and Goode 2008).

My questionnaire built on earlier research in that it included all the questions previously asked in a questionnaire designed by Glen Wilson and David Cox, administered to members of the London-based Paedophile Information Exchange (PIE) and published in *The Child-Lovers: A Study of Paedophiles in*

Society (1983). However, Wilson and Cox were psychologists and their study included a personality test component which this study avoided.

Alongside some basic demographic data, questions were asked which aimed to tease out how individuals had developed their self-identity as paedophile, what had contributed to that identity formation, how their immediate social circle responded, and where they derived support for their self-esteem and for making decisions about their behaviour. The questions also aimed to explore their views about issues such as sexual contact with children, age of consent, use of child pornography, child sex tourism, and child protection. I was also interested in finding out more about how they felt about relationships and friendships with children. In addition, there were questions about their religious affiliation, and the final part of the questionnaire explored their experiences and views on the relationship between the 'paedophile community' and ordinary society. The final question asked, 'Are there any other questions I should have asked you, or any other information you would like me to know?' At the end of the questionnaire was the opportunity for the respondent to indicate whether they agreed to stay in touch and answer further questions. The questionnaires were emailed back to me, either directly by the respondent or indirectly by way of the 'participant coordinators group'. Some respondents, trusting neither myself nor the 'participant coordinators group' but nevertheless keen to participate, set up temporary anonymous email addresses to return the questionnaires. A surprising number of respondents opted to remain in touch and continued to answer questions.

As the data came in, I removed any identifying information from the questionnaire and printed out only one single copy which was then stored securely in a locked container. I then emailed back to thank the participant, confirm that I had received their questionnaire safely and confirm also that I would now delete the email and any soft copies of the information. If they had agreed to stay in touch, I confirmed this with them. By the end of the project, all that remained therefore was one single paper copy of each completed questionnaire. I had communicated with around sixty-two self-defined paedophiles (both anonymous and 'out'), including authors, academics, and web-editors of the most influential paedophile sites on the Internet. I had conducted two taped interviews and received seventy-seven completed questionnaires in total from fifty-seven respondents (including preliminary, main and follow-up questionnaires). Around twenty-eight individuals had remained in contact to answer further questions, expanding on the data in the main questionnaire. I had also corresponded with Perverted Justice, the major online anti-paedophile organisation and many other influential people in this area, both 'pro' and 'anti'.

The project was advertised on half a dozen websites, including the key girl-lover website. The key boy-lover website was less welcoming of the project but, after checking it out very carefully, did not block it. Other sites urged people to participate. For example, one website noted, under the heading 'Important Research Project', the following:

Paul Fisher (a trusted member of our community) and Dr Sarah Goode (a respected sociologist) are currently running a research project, with the intention of enabling society to understand people who are sexually attracted to minors. This study is important for us, as the anonymity it provides should lead to much participation from non-offenders, as opposed to the contact offenders who are usually sampled by researchers in unrepresentative prison studies.

Another website posted up my comments to encourage people to participate:

A research project is being conducted at the University of Winchester, UK, on an 'internet-based sample of individuals who are sexually attracted to children or adolescents', and seeks to 'gather reliable data from this population, and to publish the results and conclusions drawn from the data ethically and impartially'.

The lead researcher is Dr. Sarah Goode, Programme Director of the Community Development Programme at the University of Winchester. In a personal statement to prospective participants, Dr. Goode says:

'I believe this research is a unique opportunity to see the world from the perspective of the paedophile. My intention is that this project will be able to counter the current hysteria around paedophilia, which helps no one. Given that perhaps 2 per cent of all men (and a smaller proportion of women) experience this preference, we urgently need to develop our understanding so that, as a society, we can make rational, informed and evidence-based decisions.'

A central issue of the project was the reaction to it by the online paedophile community, without whose interest and support there would have been no research, and this is now addressed in the following section.

Section II: The responses of the 'paedophile community' to the project

I relied entirely on the goodwill of the 'paedophile community' to advertise the project and provide data. This was a strange feeling of loss of control, as all the work I put into the project was dependent for its outcome on people whom I had typically never met and whom I knew, if at all, generally only through emails and pseudonyms. By the end of the project, I had actually met or spoken by telephone with just six people whose attitudes to the project were crucial. Of those six, I only knew the real names of three of them. At the same time, there was a clear sense that much correspondence was going on about the project to which I was not party.

Thus, it was very difficult for me to assess how the paedophile community felt about this research. Doubtless most conversations about the project were carried on either by telephone or through Internet channels which were not open to the public. I also did not make efforts to track any discussions, or in any way 'argue my case', as I felt it was better to maintain a low profile and just see what happened. The risk in 'arguing my case' would have been that I would have been repeatedly challenged and questioned on my own personal stance (for example, how did I feel about sexual contact between adults and children? Was I against it in all cases or did I agree that it might be okay under some circumstances?). These were the sorts of questions I strongly wanted to avoid having to answer, especially in a public forum, as I was clear in my own mind that I would not lie if asked a direct question, and would attempt to answer as honestly and openly as possible, but any statement of views on my part would be bound to alienate at least some members of the 'paedophile community' and therefore would be counterproductive in recruiting respondents from as wide a range of viewpoints as possible.

I was also very keen to avoid any situation where I 'led people on' and, perhaps even inadvertently, led them to expect that my personal view, and therefore my research analysis, would be more sympathetic to their position than in fact was the case. I did not want anyone to feel disappointed, cheated, or betrayed after having participated in this research. It was therefore extremely important to word all my communications very carefully, to present an even-handed approach which did not alienate anyone but at the same time did not hold out a false promise that I agreed with any particular position.

This is quite a difficult feat to achieve and, as the ethics approval for the project dragged on for what felt like endless years, this made it even harder to maintain such a carefully judged, neutral, bland stance, trying never to present a comment which could be taken out of context and used to argue that I held one position or another. It was therefore a deliberate policy on my part to keep quiet and simply allow community members themselves to argue for or against participating in this project. There were only two situations in which I was unable to avoid presenting any information publicly (other than through the Information Sheet and Questionnaire). The first situation occurred because the MAA website was revised, to encourage more participation, and I was asked to write a piece from my own perspective. I was reluctant to do this, and involved one particular respondent, 'Bernard', as a community member, to write something. In the end, two personal statements were written and published on the website, towards the end of 2007, one from myself and one from Paul Fisher.

The homepage of the website included the following, written by Paul:

> Welcome to the Minor-attracted Adult Research Project website. This funded study seeks to conduct research on an internet-based sample of individuals who are sexually attracted to children or adolescents. Most studies of such individuals have been based on prison or clinical samples, rather than those who simply self-identify as being sexually attracted to youth. This project seeks to gather reliable data from this population, and to publish the results and conclusions drawn from the data ethically and impartially.

Paul also included information about the university and myself, taken from the university webpages, including the fact that I was at that time running an undergraduate programme in community development:

> We all need our communities to work well together, and Community Development hopes to provide the theory and the practical tools to achieve this. It is a growing field, actively involved in local communities, and seeking both to help solve community problems and strengthening our democracy. This focus of Dr. Goode's work is salient to minor-attracted people, who may feel alienated from the power structures of society and true political participation in the West.

Paul then explained the role of the 'participant coordinators group':

> This research project is being conducted by Dr. Goode in collaboration with participant coordinators (in social science terminology, research gatekeepers), individuals who experience sexual attraction to youth and have responsibility to publicise the project in venues that would attract participation by eligible research participants, and also responsibility for liaising with research respondents.
>
> This website, and its content, are the work product of the participant coordinators. Dr. Goode retains copyright to her work that is reproduced here from the public domain, and to her letter addressed to potential participants, reproduced here. Dr. Goode has full responsibility for the research. Participant coordinators do not have a formal role other than as research gatekeepers. Completed research questionnaires should be returned directly to Dr. Goode at her University e-mail address (see contact). Participant coordinators can arrange a secure e-mail account for you, if you wish, for secure correspondence with the research team.

The homepage of the website concluded:

> If you are a person who experiences sexual attraction to youth, we hope you will consider participating in this study and completing the research questionnaire. Your effort is valuable. A discussion of issues that have been raised in the early phases of this research is available in our Frequently Asked Questions. If you are ready to complete the questionnaire, please feel free to choose a method of responding that is most convenient to you. The research team simply needs to know which question you are answering, and response can be in the form of a text file, email, Adobe PDF file, or Microsoft Word file.

This was followed by a FAQ section and copies of the Information Sheet and the Questionnaire for participants to complete. There were also links to a statement by myself and a statement by Paul.

Writing my statement for posting publicly on the Internet (where I knew it would be seen by paedophiles from every political and philosophical persuasion, as well as by anti-paedophile activists) was not easy. I knew it needed to be as bland and non-controversial as possible. I also knew it needed to be easily readable by those whose first language was not English. I wanted it to be entirely honest. I also wanted to encourage participation from as wide a range of participants as possible. I kept my statement as brief and neutral as I could and, before sending it off, I confirmed with the police that it was not illegal and was unlikely to be construed as advocating or inciting illegal activity.

RESEARCHER'S STATEMENT

Dear Potential Research Participant,

My name is Dr. Sarah Goode, and I am a sociologist. My previous research has concerned mothers who were drug or alcohol-dependent. I explored what it meant for those women to be labelled as 'junkies' or 'alcoholics', and how those around them responded.

My interest is in the ways in which individuals and communities develop and deal with stigmatised and hidden identities. I am also interested in how communities (especially online communities) can work to support individuals.

I believe this research is a unique opportunity to see the world from the perspective of the paedophile. My intention is that this project will be able to counter the current hysteria around paedophilia, which helps no one. Given that perhaps 2 per cent of all men (and a smaller proportion of women) experience this preference, we urgently need to develop our understanding so that, as a society, we can make rational, informed and evidence-based decisions.

Sincerely,

Sarah Goode, Ph.D.

Paul Fisher wrote a much lengthier statement to explain his interest in the research project, and his own philosophy on paedophilia. He reminded readers that individuals from the paedophile community, including Tom O'Carroll, had previously liaised with two academic researchers and he included the comments:

Twenty-five years ago, Tom O'Carroll worked with David Cox and Glen Wilson to conduct research similar to this project on the Pedophile Information Exchange (PIE) membership. The Daily Lives project includes all of the original Cox questions, but is not employing any personality test component. Tom secured seventy-seven responses for the Cox research team from the membership of PIE, and the research results were published in book format, *The Child-Lovers: A Study of Paedophiles in Society,* London: Peter Owen Publishers (1983).

I am involved in this research project because I think it is important at this time to open the door to a cultural, or sociological, perspective of minor attraction as a legitimate avenue of research inquiry. ... I believe also that in the past there existed a 'pedophile culture', long since lost to the ravages of wind and rain, and I hope to understand in this lifetime what my culture is.

...Early in this research project, I worked with others in my community to determine if Dr. Goode's proposed project would be conducted in a fair and impartial manner, or whether it was an attempt to legitimate a fraudulent research finding. I have confidence in Sarah. She has had broad life-experiences involving other counter- or sub-cultural groups, such as her squatting with punks, rockers and radical queer activists in North London, hanging out with a Gypsy family on the banks of the Loire River (and very nearly eating snails), spending a year as a Buddhist nun, and spending time helping rehabilitate children in Bethlehem, including spinal-injured teenagers who had been shot during the Intifada.

The information about my life, quoted here by Paul, was taken from a biographical note I had written and posted on my university website before commencing this research project. Paul has considerately not included the information – also given in the biographical note – that I am a mother of young children. The full biographical note reads:

I joined King Alfred's (now the University of Winchester) in April 2001, after a year investigating disability issues at the University of Warwick, where I also previously completed an MA and PhD in medical sociology.

Before that I qualified and worked as an occupational therapist. Generally speaking, before that I had various interesting life experiences, including squatting with punks, rockers and radical queer activists in North London, travelling around free festivals with Willi X and The Convoy, hanging out with a Gypsy family on the banks of the Loire River (and very nearly eating snails), spending a year as a Buddhist nun, and spending time helping rehabilitate children in Bethlehem, including spinal-injured teenagers who had been shot during the Intifada. I have also worked as a chambermaid, a cook in a police station, a shop assistant in an occult bookshop, a mail-order philately clerk (believe me, philately will get you nowhere), an assembly line night-worker in a plastics factory, and a clerk-typist for a loan-shark company. In addition, I've done respite fostering for a young boy with cerebral palsy, and fostered a 14-year-old mother and her newborn. I've also done boring things but I can't remember them offhand.

My interests are trying to understand the world we live in, particularly people, and I have two children who help me very much in my academic work, by joining in whenever I try to type anything on the computer, and by interrupting me every time I try to read.

I was astonished to think that my involvement with political squats in north London in 1979 had smoothed the way for me, almost thirty years later, to research online paedophiles! When I wrote my biographical note, choosing those aspects of my life to highlight, my intention had been to present myself to my students as someone friendly and approachable. A year later, I had in fact updated and amended it to make it much more sober and 'normal', but for some reason this update had not replaced the old version. Several years later, this random oversight appeared to make a major difference to the success of this project.

Paul knew at the time that he wrote this endorsement that he was taking a risk of it backfiring. As someone with high visibility within the paedophile community, he was risking his reputation as a trusted and knowledgeable individual by publicly naming himself as involved in this project. The whole project therefore hung on his credibility within the MAA community. He devoted considerable time arguing the case for this project, and answering criticisms. I was only vaguely aware of any of this going on. I only knew when some of the arguments spilled out past Paul and affected me directly. For example, in September 2007 I was telephoned on my mobile, out of the blue, by the web editor of a major pro-paedophile website. Apparently, this individual had been involved in long conversations about the project after he had objected to an announcement about the project being posted on his site. As he explained, 'We're the big guys – we are where journos go when they want to find out what paedophiles are up to.' As the key person involved with security on this major website, his concern seemed to be mainly that my research would necessitate revealing my sources and so he needed to check me out. He remained fairly sceptical and decided he would not in any way endorse my research by suggesting to people that they should participate, but after communicating with me, he was happy for details to remain posted on the website.

As can be seen from this overview of my interactions with the 'paedophile community', I had to tread very carefully throughout the duration of the research and I relied heavily on the goodwill of various individuals, to whom I remain sincerely grateful for their courteous support.

5   Findings from the Minor-Attracted Adults Daily Lives Research Project

I recently heard the ecologist and environmentalist Michael Tobias talking about the disaster that awaits the human race if we don't get our population growth under control. He...described the necessary approach as requiring 'restraint, gentleness and grace'. It struck me that these are qualities I try to emphasise in my attempts to advocate for myself and others like me, and are also at the core of my practical ethos with kids, especially if I have strong feelings for them. I think I'm talking to you now because I think you demonstrate these qualities. I understand that aspects of my orientation might upset and disturb you and others, and I've had some painful conflicts with my own friends, but I think if people try to develop mutual respect and have patience, things get easier. The small amount of tolerance and understanding I've been shown by a few people in my life have made me much more open to the concerns and anxieties people have around this subject. Which must be a good thing, surely.

(Tim)

Introduction

This chapter presents information from a sample of fifty-six self-defined pae-dophiles, who have all volunteered information on their everyday lives and their views and experiences on how it feels to live as an adult sexually attracted to children.

Some participants were so enthusiastic about this project that they wrote questionnaire responses running into many thousands of words: 15,000 words was probably the longest response but several others were of similar length. In addition, a number stayed in contact for weeks, months or even years, writing innumerable and lengthy emails detailing their experiences, thoughts and the intimate details of their sexual feelings. A number of correspondents sent a dozen or more emails: one, who was a key player in the research, sent over 120 emails over the course of the project, almost all of them thoughtful and intel-lectually engaged and all of them unfailingly courteous. (At times these made a refreshing contrast to the emails I received from more 'mainstream' sources.) Two lengthy taped interviews were also conducted. By the end of the research I felt somewhat overwhelmed by the volume and depth of information.

Breaking down this mass of information into readable accounts has been quite a task, especially since I kept only hard copies (print-outs) of the questionnaire responses and deleted soft copies for security. Therefore, all analysis has been conducted manually rather than using software and all quotations have been typed out by hand. This slowed the process of analysis but helped me to become more familiar with each questionnaire response and the flow of respondents' accounts.

The preliminary, pilot, questionnaire was circulated and completed by eight respondents in 2006. Subsequently, the questionnaire was revised and expanded, using feedback and suggestions from a number of people within the online paedophile community and also advice from academic and professional colleagues. It was circulated during the second half of 2007 and was completed by fifty-one respondents in total (five of whom had also completed the pilot); thus fifty-four respondents in total sent me completed questionnaires, either preliminary or main. Twenty-eight respondents indicated that they would be happy to answer further questions as these emerged from the data-analysis. Not all of these could be followed up, as some email addresses had expired. However, eighteen did complete follow-up further questions and others answered additional questions or discussed further issues. At the end of the data collection, therefore, I had received a total of seventy-seven questionnaires (eight preliminary, fifty-one main and eighteen follow-up) from fifty-four respondents. I also had two recorded interviews. (I received a completed questionnaire from one respondent which is not included in the analysis, as it was written by someone aged seventeen who described himself as sexually attracted to adult men. He discussed a current relationship with an adult man he had met online and with whom he had had a sexual relationship for 'three years or more', in other words since he was aged under fourteen. This information might have been useful if it had been expanded and if there had been information provided by other 'loved boys' but as it was not the primary focus of this research and contained only minimal information this questionnaire had to be deleted from the sample.) In addition, I had also corresponded with a number of self-defined paedophiles, some of whom had not completed any formal data collection instruments but who had provided me with a great deal of background information, for example on attitudes within the online paedophile community and ways in which this community works.

The main questionnaire collected information on approximately sixty different elements, with almost all the questions providing the opportunity for text-based answers of whatever length the respondent wished. By the end of the data collection, therefore, I had well over 1,000 separate pieces of information provided for analysis, with some items being discussed in great detail over several pages, and thus many tens of thousands of words of raw data. (As I write this, I am also still receiving emails from respondents staying in touch to comment on my work.) Not all of this data can be fully presented here, and some topics have had to be left out of this discussion. Hopefully, future publications will be able to remedy some of these omissions. Where topics have been discussed in this book, I have attempted as far as practical to provide full quotations from all the respondents. Where this is not possible, quotations have been chosen to be generally representative of the types of responses given.

In all cases, the pseudonyms given in this study are ones chosen by me. Some respondents offered pseudonyms that they would like me to use, or even gave me permission to use their actual names, but I was careful to explain that these would not be used in this study as I needed to ensure the highest level of anonymity. A distribution of English and non-English names have been used to reflect the spread of nationalities among the respondents, but individual pseudonyms do not reflect the actual nationality of the individual respondent. It is possible that, where a respondent is particularly well known in a community, more than one pseudonym has been used by me, to further reduce the likelihood of identifying a person from biographical details. In some cases the English has been corrected for clarity and to reduce the possibility of identification by non-standard English usage. In all cases, the spelling of 'paedophile' has been given using the British convention.

Section I of this chapter introduces the respondents, outlining the basic demographic details of gender, nationality, age and other characteristics. Section II begins the process of exploring the data, looking at respondents' own sexual experiences as children; their experiences of marriage and parenthood; and their contact with the law. The following chapters then pick up the issues of identity, fantasy, support and the differing views expressed by the respondents.

Section I: Basic demographic details of sample

> As I found myself examining every last girl that walked by, I finally admitted to myself that without doubt I was attracted to children.
>
> (Kristof)

(A) Gender

Of the fifty-six respondents, all but two are male. This low rate of response from women occurred despite my urging gatekeepers to encourage women in particular to participate. Three of the sample were aged under twenty-one years, and wherever these respondents are quoted their age is given in brackets, to distinguish them from all the other respondents.

(B) Nationality and ethnicity

In giving their responses to my questions, there were many quirky and often witty answers. For example, not everyone appreciated being asked for demographic data about nationality and in response to the question, 'Please give your nationality and ethnicity', one person wrote: '"Ethnicity" is a fallacy, and comprises a tiny insignificant fraction of the genetic differences among humans.

May as well ask my astrological sign, which is just as identifying, and just as irrelevant.' See Table 5.1 for the countries and ethnic identities named by the respondents.

(C) Language

This emphasis on the North American experience reflects the fact that English-language pro-paedophile sites are often, although not exclusively, associated with the USA, and that at present ownership of personal computers is higher in the USA than in most other countries (for example, see Shah 2007). The 'paedophile community' is a community without geographical boundaries, where influential ideas circulate easily within and between countries. A number of pro-paedophile websites have multiple-language web-pages, so their influence is not restricted to English-speakers only: this project, however, researched only the English-language component of these sites and communities.

Of the fifty-six respondents, eleven did not have English as a first language but their written English was still of a generally high standard, allowing them to express themselves competently. A reasonable level of ability in written English was required to understand and respond to the questions, therefore the respondents were self-selected in terms of fluency as well as access to the Internet. As far as I am aware, the questionnaire was publicised only on English-language sites.

(D) Age

The bulk of the respondents are aged from twenty-one to thirty, with another nine aged from thirty-one to forty. Only three respondents were aged younger than twenty-one, with the remainder aged from their forties up to their seventies. See Table 5.2 for the age ranges of the respondents.

This age-distribution is what one would expect from an Internet-based sample, which tends to reflect the age of those people most attracted to Internet use, who

Table 5.1 Countries involved

Country	Number of respondents
North America (USA and Canada)	28
United Kingdom	8
Other European	7
Australasia (Australia and New Zealand)	5
Netherlands	5
Other ('White', 'Caucasian')	3
Total	**56**

Table 5.2 Age of respondents

Age	Number of respondents
Younger than 21	3
21 to 30	24
31 to 40	16
41 and older	13
Total	**56**

are usually in their twenties and thirties. The older respondents tended to be people who have been active within the 'paedophile community' for a number of years.

It also reflects the fact that it was stipulated that respondents should be aged over twenty-one years to participate in the research (see Chapter 3, Section III). This stipulation was included because it was felt by one commentator (Professor Richard Green) that it was common for individuals aged under twenty-one years to be sexually attracted to people aged under sixteen years old. Even if true, this factor was unlikely to influence the findings of the research because, in order to participate, an individual would need to be visiting pro-paedophile websites and also would need to self-identify as sexually attracted to minors themselves – which many people would be loath to do. However, it was included as a stipulation. This also avoided the potential ethical difficulty of soliciting information from those aged under the age of majority (eighteen years in the USA, sixteen years in the UK), in which case permission would need to be sought from their parent or guardian before they could participate in the research.

Unknown to me, this stipulation provoked an angry response on websites where the research was advertised. Some potential respondents felt excluded and unable to contribute and engaged in heated and extensive dialogue about this with the Project Coordinator. When I found out that this had occurred, I explained to the Coordinator about the ethics restriction on soliciting information. In the event, four individuals aged under twenty-one years volunteered information (of whom one, as mentioned, was in a sexual relationship with an older man, was not himself sexually attracted to children, and was thus excluded). The information from the other three respondents (Ed, Freddy and Ulf) has been included in the analysis of the data. It would seem to be a mark of the honesty of respondents that, rather than give a false age, they preferred to protest and to complete the questionnaire giving what appears to be their true age, even where they were unsure that, having done so, their data would then be accepted. Their data has been used, but in each case where they are quoted, their age is shown in brackets.

(E) Educational level

This small sample included a spread of educational levels including graduate, postgraduate and doctorate level, and occupations included, for example, teacher, academic, religious minister, computer programmer, truck-driver, store-manager and unemployed.

(F) Orientation of attraction

Oddly, the sample was equally divided between people sexually attracted to boys (twenty-four) and girls (twenty-four), with the remainder (eight) finding both attractive. Neither the gatekeepers nor I could have controlled this distribution, so it was surprising and interesting that it worked out to contain exactly equal numbers of 'girl-lovers' and 'boy-lovers'. This was despite the fact that the project was almost certainly advertised more energetically on a major 'girl-lover' site than on the equivalent 'boy-lover' site. This greater advertising to 'girl-lovers' may have overcome the possibly greater preponderance of 'boy-lovers' on the Internet in general, but this is speculative and would need further research to validate.

(G) Length of time respondents had been sexually attracted to children

The age-distribution of the sample, shown above, has a relationship with experience. Not all respondents were asked how long they had known they were sexually attracted to children but, of the thirty-seven about whom this information is known, the distribution divides up rather neatly and symmetrically: only five had been aware of their attraction for less than ten years (usually around five years); fourteen had known for ten or more years; and eighteen had known for twenty or more years, including five with experience going back more than thirty years. The sample therefore, despite being skewed towards those in their twenties and thirties, included a substantial number of individuals with a long period of relevant experience to draw on in their responses. See Table 5.3 for information on how long respondents had been sexually attracted to children.

(H) Process of first becoming aware of sexual attraction to children

Becoming aware of their sexual attraction to children was described by many as a gradual process. As they entered puberty, they found themselves sexually awakening and attracted to same-age peers, then gradually noticing that their 'age of attraction' remained fairly static while they themselves grew older. For many, as with David whom we met in Chapter 1, this was a slow process of bewilderment, shock, denial and eventual acceptance. The process of first recognition of their sexual attraction tended to happen between the ages of eleven up to their late teens, although seven respondents described it as occurring while they were themselves aged ten or younger and for two or three respondents sexual attraction to children or young people seems to have developed only in full adulthood, in their thirties or beyond.

> *I came to full realisation of what my sexual attractions were when I was about twelve. But looking back on my life, I realise I always knew, going all the way back to kindergarten.*
>
> (Gus)

> *Since my earliest youth...Vague knowing before the age of ten, conscious knowing about the age of thirteen, even more conscious from the age of seventeen.*
>
> (Pete)

> *I knew it very soon, although I didn't know the word for it. I think I was aware of it around my thirteenth.*
>
> (Oscar)

> *In some ways I've been attracted to them since I was their age. ... I didn't really think anything odd about it at the time, and I still don't know how 'normal' it is for young teenage boys to be attracted to girls a few years younger. It never really bothered me, though. As I approached my twenties, however, my feelings began to disturb me. I thought it might be a phase or the product of sexual frustration. Whatever it was, I didn't like it, and I began to feel awful about myself. If I had to point to a single moment of realisation, it would be a temporary summer job that I held one year. I wasn't used to being around children, but here they were all over. It was outside in the heat, so the clothing was revealing. As I found myself examining every last girl that walked by, I finally admitted to myself that without doubt I was attracted to children.*
>
> (Kristof)

> *It wasn't until I was thirty and had my first love affair with a young boy that I had my epiphany: that I wasn't a heterosexual with a quirky attraction to boys, but rather a boylover, lying to myself for many years.*
>
> (Jerry)

Table 5.3 Length of time respondents had been sexually attracted to children

Age	Number of respondents
Less than 10 years	5
Between 10 and 20 years	14
Between 20 and 30 years	13
Over 30 years	5
Total	**37**

Section II: Experiences related to sexuality

I've loved 'sex play' since childhood.

(Tim)

It will be remembered that no questions were asked which could incriminate respondents and thus no respondent was asked about sexual experiences as an adult with a child. However, respondents were asked about sexual experiences which they had had when they themselves were children. Respondents also wrote about their relationships with adults and briefly mentioned their own experiences as parents. (They were also asked about their attitudes to sex with adults and this is dealt with in the following chapter.) In terms of how they dealt with their sexuality, respondents were asked about any contact with the law and the impact this had had on them.

(A) First sexual experience

Forty-six of the fifty-six respondents were asked about their first sexual experiences (not all used the versions which contained this question). Of those who were asked, two declined to answer this question, one stated 'I have not had physical sexual interactions with others'; one described a subjectively erotic experience which had no physical sexual component (skating with a small child when he was aged eleven); one gave his earliest sexual experience as occurring at age ten but did not describe the experience, and another reported he had 'flashed' (exposed his genitals) when at school, but gave no age for this. In addition, one reported an experience of forced sexual contact:

> *Forced, when I was around six, by a man. My memory of it is unclear and probably inaccurate.*

(Freddy, aged sixteen)

Since the other experiences were not reported as forced, this experience is taken as qualitatively different. Thus, of the forty-six who were asked, thirty-nine provided answers which gave information on age at first sexual experience and which were not described as forced. The topic of 'first sexual experience' is of course one which is difficult to define and sometimes difficult to recall. To the question, 'Describe the earliest sexual experience you can remember', people responded by describing the age at which they first masturbated or the age at which they first 'played doctor' or 'made out'. In future questionnaires, it might be useful to ask specifically about first experience of masturbation and first experience with another person. Nevertheless, the question produced some unexpected findings.

Of the thirty-nine responses dealing with direct sexual experiences where sufficient information was given, three were referred to as first occurring when the respondent was aged eighteen, twenty and twenty-one years old. Of the remaining thirty-six, all had occurred before the age of fourteen.

Thirty-two of these experiences occurred when the respondent was aged twelve or under, and only four when the respondent was aged thirteen or fourteen. Nine respondents referred to masturbation as their earliest sexual experience, with two respondents describing memories of masturbating from the age of three or four; two from the age of six; two from the age of seven to eight; and three from between eleven to thirteen. (Three respondents reported orgasm from masturbation starting at six, eight and nine years of age.) Twenty-one respondents reported their earliest sexual experience as sex play with an approximately same-age peer, with two respondents reporting sex play from the age of three or four; six from ages five or six; eight from ages seven to nine; two from ages eleven and twelve, and three when they were aged thirteen or fourteen. In addition, one reported contact with a younger child when he was aged seven, and five reported contact with an older person or adult when they were aged from five to eight years old. As with any retrospective data, it is necessary to be cautious about these reports. For example, two respondents gave two different accounts of their earliest sexual experiences.

> *[First account] Masturbation at age fourteen. [Second account] At age eleven years I participated in group masturbatory experiments with other boys and played 'I'll show you mine if you show me yours' with the girl next door.*
>
> (Nigel)

> *[First account] It was an older boy from the neighbourhood who was twelve and I was like seven or so and we masturbated each other and body rubbed. [Second account] I was a young boy when I was sexually active with my uncle when I was around five or six.*
>
> (Ian)

[In both these cases the second account is the one used in analysis. It may be of course that in the second example the uncle was aged twelve and lived in the neighbourhood.]

Despite treating individual accounts with caution, what emerges from this cumulative data are a picture, not of individuals who were sexually abused as children but individuals who were sexually active as children, often from a young age. Again, the question on 'earliest sexual experience' obscures the situations when the experience might have been a very mild single occasion or a particularly memorable episode within an ongoing pattern. Examples of responses include:

> *When I was about seven I felt the chest of an approximately four-year-old girl.*
>
> (Oliver)

I and my brothers became friends with one girl. Anyway, after a year or so (aged around eight) I walked into my room and my brothers were playing 'doctor'. They asked if I would like to join. I declined. I didn't want to get in trouble if we were caught. I don't know if you count that as a sexual experience, I do because it was the first time I saw a girl naked.

(Stewart)

Early sexual expression or experimentation was my friend Chris who was four, and I who was five, played with each other's penises. My first sexual orgasmic experience was two weeks into my tenth birthday masturbating to pictures of other youths or adults from magazines and so on.

(Ralph)

At age eight I had anal sex with same age. ... I continued to have sex from age seven on. I showed a neighbour boy who was about six and we started sex almost every day for the next seven or eight years. I also had many others I was having sex with in the neighbourhood as well, not all initiated by me. Either from some other adults to teenagers to preteen. Whoever was willing or wanted to play we did it with them.

(Max)

Masturbating by myself to orgasm by rubbing my crotch on a shimmy pole on a playground when I was six. I learned how to do it on my own.

(Justin)

I played doctor with a female playmate at my home when I was five years old.

(Clive)

I remember playing 'doctor' type games with many young children, male and female, from about the age of five. I would often spend the night with two neighbouring sisters and we would often engage in sex play at night in bed.

(Jerry)

'Playing doctor' with a peer of the same age at age eight.

(Derek)

Truth or dare with friends around nine or something, from touching up to blowjobs.

(Hugo)

I was about eight years old. A male neighbour (about fourteen at the time) engaged me in oral sex. I found it very enjoyable and exciting. ... The oral sex continued for a number of years. I was never forced. Several times my neighbour asked me to return the favour but the sight of his hair was particularly off-putting to me and I never did it.

(Louis)

A neighbour boy and I compared ourselves to each other and touched each other at age six. First actual sex at age thirteen to fourteen when I seduced and performed oral sex on a eleven- to twelve-year-old neighbour.

(Hans)

The earliest sexual experience was with my best friend when we were about nine or ten. It lasted until about twelve when the spectre of homosexuality made its presence felt and it just stopped.

(John)

Underwear fetish/self play at age three – as early as I can remember. Genital showing with female at age seven – slight contact between genitals. Masturbation to orgasm at age nine.

(Wayne)

See Table 5.4 for data on the reported earliest sexual experience for the thirty-six respondents about whom this data is known.

In this small and non-random sample, therefore, there is little to support the posited 'cycle of abuse' in which it is assumed that paedophiles were sexually abused by adults in childhood and go on to sexually abuse children in their turn (for a further discussion of this, see for example Itzin 2000). As one individual commented:

I experienced extensive sexual contact with an adult as a child (five to eight years old); many in my life have assumed my orientation derives from that incident. I do not believe so. The incidence of sexual contact with

Table 5.4 Figures for reported earliest sexual experience

Age	Solo masturbation	Peer sex play	Younger peer	Older peer	Adult	Total
Earliest sexual experience age 3–6	4	8		1	1	**14**
Earliest sexual experience age 7–9	2	8	1	1	2	**14**
Earliest sexual experience age 10–12	2	2				**4**
Earliest sexual experience age 13–14	1	3				**4**
Total	**9**	**21**	**1**	**2**	**3**	**36**

adults as minors, within the population of minor-attracted adults, seems to parallel fairly closely that statistic for 'straight' society. I participated in 'survivors' (an American term popular for sexual abuse victims) groups for many years, always fully upfront about my sexual issues. I had a deep understanding of both sides of that token. I carry no sensitivities in discussing that topic; I felt anger at one point towards the man I was sexually involved with, and have resolved it over the years.

Rather than the emphasis on abuse by adults, there is a suggestion of sexually interested and active children who explore their own and other children's bodies out of curiosity and pleasure. To what extent this sample may vary from the general population in the age and amount of early sexual exploration is unclear, but childish games of exploratory sexuality such as 'playing doctor' or discovering masturbation seem fairly widespread: for example, see Levine (2002) and, from a literary perspective, the autobiographical accounts by the writer Blake Morrison (1997 and 2002). What may distinguish this sample more clearly from the general population is perhaps that they may grow up to retain into their adulthood their continuing sexual curiosity in 'playing doctor' or 'show me yours and I'll show you mine'.

It's clear to me in hindsight that as I went through puberty I grew increasingly nostalgic for girls as equals, with the physical confidence they had as preadolescents. ... I was basically a stranger to adulthood, and I still am. ... it's possible I'm 'attuned' to children because something within me is still a child. ... there is an immediate recognition of [childlike qualities] that I can trace unbroken to my own childhood. I have always felt this way. I think perhaps I am different not because I feel them but because I have not ceased to feel them. ... I've loved 'sex play' since childhood. ... The earliest consciously sexual solo experience I can remember is taking off my pants and humping the [fur] rug on my bed. I can clearly remember pushing my erection through the fur and it feeling very nice. It was connected with nap time, so I must have been six at the most. ... I really enjoyed sex play with girls in my childhood. Games typically involved some privacy, some close inspection of bottoms and genitals and maybe insertion of a button or pencil or a finger. ... my sister grassed on me for examining her vulva (she was about seven, I was about nine). I was punished somehow and felt it very unfair and ran away from home for a day. ... I was quite interested in girlfriends at this age. ... When I was eleven or so, I formed quite a romantic attachment with a little girl of six or seven during the holidays, and we exchanged letters for a while...The friendship attracted some amused comment. ... By the time I left [school] at eighteen, I had lost all of that ease. ... Girls my own age didn't intimidate me exactly, but they seemed matronly in a way I found sexually uninteresting. I knew I was sexually interested in young girls by that time. I fantasised about them and felt guilty and ashamed about it. ... By the time I left school I was

*drinking enough to black out most weekends, practically an alcoholic. ... I
was frustrated. I got more and more wound up and anxious until I couldn't
make head or tail of any of it. It's been like that ever since. All I ever
really wanted was a soulmate.*

(Tim)

(B) Marriage and parenthood

As well as being sexually attracted to children, some respondents also found
themselves attracted to adults – or had attempted to have sexual relationships
with adults in order to 'pass' as normal. This is dealt with in the following
chapter, as part of the examination of respondents' self-identities. What is
significant to note here, in terms of a family life, is that at least five and
possibly more of the respondents had at some point been married (only
twenty-three of the respondents were asked this question), and six of the
respondents had children, with another whose wife was pregnant at the time
of completing the questionnaire. In addition, one respondent felt that they
had been regarded as an informal parent-figure by many children and two
respondents answered that they hoped to be parents in the future.

Thus, of a sample of fifty-one (five respondents were not asked this question),
over one in ten of the respondents reported that they were parents. At least
one of the parents had also been a foster-parent and was now a grandparent.
This response rate is perhaps particularly significant given that a member of
the community noted that it would be more difficult and unlikely for a parent
or someone with custodial responsibility for children to access and complete
the questionnaire. This is because they would be likely to be much more
cautious about investigating paedophile-related Internet sites, both because of
legal repercussions on their parental status if discovered, and also practically
because in a shared household it was more likely that other people might discover
what they were looking at. Thus a rate of around 10 per cent, in this sample,
indicates that men who are parents may make up a significant sub-group within
those who self-define as paedophile.

*I have had sex with adults (my ex-wife mainly), and am [a] father [...]. Sex
with my wife was usually good, often very good. I almost always fantasised
that she was a child, and she often helped me by dressing as a schoolgirl.
Sex with my wife was most satisfying when I successfully fantasised about her
being a child.*

(Lenny)

*I 'believe' that sex is for male and female within the context of a marriage.
However, personally I find the idea of sex with females to be very distasteful, even nauseating, adult females particularly so. Despite this, I have
been married to a female adult for about twenty years. I have engaged*

sexually by leaning heavily on boy fantasy during sex. Without the fantasy, I cannot maintain arousal. ... the idea of pubic hair is particularly off putting to me.

(Louis)

This issue of sexual attraction, fantasy and desire will be examined in the next chapter, and the question of support by family members is also addressed later. In terms of actual behaviour, having experienced sexual attraction to children for somewhere between five and over sixty years, how had these men coped?

(C) Contact with the criminal justice system

The question was asked, 'Do you have any criminal convictions or police cautions relating to your sexual attraction to children? If you do, what impact has this had on your life?' (It was explained in a note at the end of the questionnaire what a 'police caution' meant, for those respondents who were not based in the UK.) This question was not asked in the preliminary questionnaire or in one of the interviews, so information was not available on this for five respondents. For the remaining fifty-one respondents, ten had had some contact with the police and the rest (forty-one) had not. The respondents were not asked what offence they were charged with, and most did not volunteer details of either the offence or the sentence. In four of the ten cases, the case had been withdrawn, set aside, acquitted or not brought to court, so that in only six cases did the respondent actually have a full criminal conviction. The sentences for these six offences included imprisonment in two cases (Ralph and Jerry), with the other sentences involving mandatory therapy, community service, probation and/or registration as a sex offender. Only one respondent (Lenny) referred to more than one conviction.

I have two convictions for downloading child pornography. The first was the result of an addiction I had to collecting child pornography from the Internet. I never paid for, requested or traded any images, but I convinced myself that I would not be caught. As a result I lost my wife and was given three years' probation and five years on the SOR [Sex Offender Register]. I obviously suffered socially, losing many friends, and since then I have had to live alone.

(Lenny)

It was never an issue until Megan's Law took effect. Now I can't find work, I have been kicked out of my last three housing situations. ... I have been fired from my last three jobs because of employee concern or public concern after seeing my photo on state websites even though my jobs were not with children. It has ruined my life.

(Max)

My conviction [has] only been another form of control and consequence that has made life even more difficult than it already is. ... Such social controls I feel are counterproductive to the reintegration of paedophiles or sex offenders into the community and only instigates [sic] the flawed concept of 'protecting' children from giving or receiving sexual orgasmic pleasure with whom they choose. ... [I received] in-house treatment while in prison under a comprehensive programme for a number of years, and then post-prison, while under parole, I attended mandatory treatment once a week for a couple more years.

(Ralph)

A conviction. ... The impact of it was disastrous. I had to move to another city and keep silence for several years. The whole process, from report until the very end of my probation time took ten years of my life.

(Pete)

I have had a few sexual contacts with two little girls...having been arrested in the past I surely don't want to go through that terrorism again. You could say that 'society' won on that one, since they got what they wanted, their terrorism worked, I don't see many children anymore. ... I still am cautious about being alone with children because of the context I still live in, not that I would want to hurt them, but I need to keep in mind that having any kind of sexual relationship with a child right now would not be a good idea.

(Carl)

I was arrested and incarcerated for my relationship with a fourteen-year-old boy. ... I'm an RSO [registered sex offender]. I've been checked, rechecked, inspected, injected and rejected, as they say. I can't even begin to list the number of jobs I've lost because of my RSO status. I'd never bother not applying, but I'm at the point where I don't fill out applications as they are time-consuming. Instead I simply contact the hiring manager and tell them directly that I'm an RSO and ask if it's worth my time to continue the application process. Ninety-nine per cent of the time the answer is a resounding no. ... I can't even begin to state the impact this had had. It's been life-altering as you can well imagine. The areas of my life this touches on are much too many to mention. ... I went to prison. I was informed in no uncertain terms that another sexual encounter with another boy would mean a return to prison. That was all I needed to hear. It's not the only reason I wouldn't engage in such behaviour again, but it was the first, and again, the only, reason I needed. If I touch a stove and get burned, I know not to touch the stove again. Lesson learned.

(Jerry)

Charges relating to possession of 'objectionable' images were subsequently withdrawn. ... Despite having no convictions my career was destroyed and my self-esteem was extremely low.

(Nigel)

I was once convicted, but the judge later signed an order, after I'd finished some community service, that set aside the conviction. There is still a record of this and I feel I have to live in a cave.

(Quentin)

*I was acquitted...to a lot of people an acquittal means nothing – to such people it is not only guilty until proved innocent; it is also guilty **after** proved innocent. ... I have lost friends and some family members have disowned me...I am now distrustful of other people, am more withdrawn and worry about what other people who know about the accusation think about me.*

(Bill)

No, but I did get sent to the police once. I was in the swimming pool, had met two children there, and it was noticed that I had a hard-on while playing with them. I got forbidden from visiting the pool for one year. It was painful at the time, but did not have lasting effects.

(Vincent)

Thus, the data in this chapter illustrate that this sample can be characterised as largely composed of men in their twenties and thirties, of whom a small number have been married or are parents. The sample contains a spread of those attracted to boys, girls or both. Although at least thirty-two of the fifty-six respondents have been sexually attracted to children for ten years or more, only six of the sample are known to have criminal convictions, and the majority appear never to have had contact with the law. The next chapter will explore in more details these individuals' inner lives, and look at how they develop a sense of themselves as being a 'paedophile'.

6   Constructing and negotiating identities

These websites have helped me to understand my attractions to a greater extent, and to understand my place as an MAA in modern society.

(Ed, aged seventeen)

Introduction

Deciding that one is 'a paedophile', given the hugely stigmatised nature of such an identity, is a major step for anyone to take. For many, the effect is to set one apart from 'society' and from one's friends and family, who often are unaware of this secret and hidden self-identity. I was interested, in this study, in how such identities were first constructed and how, over time, they might develop and become further adjusted and negotiated, particularly in relation to both the wider culture (Hollywood films, well-known novels and so on) and the specific pro-paedophile subculture existing on the Internet.

Sexuality is a large part of self-identity, particularly perhaps in contemporary Western culture where there is a strong emphasis on sexual self-determination and sexual experience, pleasure, prowess and fulfilment. Not only is sexuality bound up with one's experience of self in that sexual pleasure is considered so central, but also – as one grows into one's twenties and thirties – there is an increasing expectation of coupledom, of settling down in a stable and committed relationship and, in time, considering parenthood. Despite radical changes in how relationships are perceived in Western culture, it is still the statistical norm for people to be married and for people to be parents. As with homosexual men and women who find themselves at odds with the mainstream emphasis on normative heterosexuality, paedophiles may feel themselves set apart from 'straight society' in relation to their attitude towards sex with their peers and in their expectations about what life is likely to hold. There is a social expectation that adults will have their closest and most intimate relationships with their sexual partner. Where people do not have a sexual partner, often they miss out on emotional warmth and comfort as well as the physical release that sex can offer. Loneliness can be compounded by feelings of failure and difference, in a social world where it can sometimes feel that 'everyone' is happily partnered except oneself. These experiences of loneliness are widely shared by many individuals at points in the life cycle (for example, widowed people will share some aspects of such isolation) but for people with a primary sexual attraction to children there is likely to be a sense of being condemned to isolation without end.

As well as the physical pleasure and emotional friendship which romantic relationships lead to, the relationships are also important in themselves, as a source of excitement, meaning and focus. The feeling of 'being in love' is not only psychologically but culturally important, with a whole greetings-card industry cashing in on the sentimentality of St Valentine's Day, the patron saint of romantic love. Wherever we turn in our daily lives, we are likely to be confronted by love songs – on the radio, on the television, in the shopping malls. Such songs can be a constant reminder of what society expects of us, of what we ourselves expect of our lives. Our contemporary Western society embraces the cultural norm that if we *want,* we *do.* No barriers should stand in the way of fulfilling our desires, our potential, our personal happiness. We are all enjoined to live the dream, be yourself, have it all, you owe it to yourself, because you're worth it. Strong cultural, popular psychological and advertising messages suggest to us that we have the right to be happy, and this is true particularly in the realm of personal relationships and sexuality. It is part of what modern Western society understands as comprising mature adulthood. Once one is an adult, then one is sexual and expected to fulfil that potential. From the teens onwards, an adult is expected to be in a sexual relationship, or recovering from one, or gearing up ready for the next one. Barriers which still exist in more traditional societies have largely been lifted in contemporary secular society. Divorced or widowed people, people within sexually unfulfilling marriages, people with disabilities – all are now expected to go out there and get sexually active if they possibly can. Even older people are not exempt. Sexual desire was traditionally seen as something that diminished as we aged, releasing people to wisdom or contemplation. Not any more: any diminution of sexual appetite or prowess is now seen as a medical condition, to be treated with hormone replacement therapy or Viagra. Thus, sex is now seen as something intrinsic to our personal and social well-being, something we are expected to do whether we are married, single, partnered, heterosexual, homosexual, bisexual, transgender, queer or any number of sexual orientations and variations. Except paedophiles. Paedophiles desire what they cannot have. How do you live your life, and build your identity, on desiring what you cannot have?

The author Quentin Crisp once remarked that he was turned off by homosexual men. He only experienced sexual desire for straight men, men who would find the idea of sex with another man revolting. He was in a 'double bind', an irresolvable dilemma arising from contradictory demands (as discussed, for example, in Bateson 1972). Paedophiles can find themselves in a similar situation. Beyond the everyday frustrations and misery of seeking sexual and emotional fulfilment, for paedophiles there is the double bind of desiring what is normatively highly valued in contemporary society – a sexual relationship – while at the same time knowing that sexual behaviour with children is normatively forbidden and illegal. This sense of 'forbidden love' can lead to despair, frustration and anger, as quotations from the respondents illustrate.

In this chapter, Section I explores a somewhat unexpected finding on the respondents' views on sex with adults. Section II then sets out the sources (books, films, individuals and websites) which respondents cited as having shaped their view of themselves. Because of the importance of websites in particular to this sample, Section III looks at this issue in detail and it is returned to again in the chapter on where respondents obtained support.

Section I: Respondents' views on sex with adults

To the question, 'How do you view the idea of sex with adults?', respondents gave a range of answers. Their views varied from finding the idea of sex with adults 'dirty' or 'disgusting', to feeling neutral about it and indeed to being enthusiastic about sexual relations with adults. See Table 6.1 for a brief summary of the respondents' views on the idea of sex with adults.

The following quotations give a sense of the breadth of variety in the respondents' answers:

I view it as a thing of nightmares.

(Freddy, aged sixteen)

Only not disgusting under the influence of drugs.

(Derek)

Dirty and intimidating.

(Xavier)

Unappealing. I have attempted it a couple of times but was never aroused and thus unable to ejaculate. There was simply no chemistry at all.

(Gary)

Table 6.1 Views on idea of sex with adults

Views	Number of respondents
Negative	17
Neutral	16
Positive	14
Question not asked	6
Answer unclear and seemed to refer to adults having sex with children	3
Total	**56**

I find the idea of sex with females to be very distasteful, even nauseating, adult females particularly so.

(Louis)

Dull.

(Quentin)

To me, the idea of sex, erotic love or romantic relations with a woman just feels as though it is in the 'wrong category'.

(William)

I view the idea of sex with adults as good, normal and healthy, but adults are kinda hairy.

(Ken)

Positively, but it is not as attractive an option as children.

(Clive)

I have a stable girlfriend of my own age and having sex with her has always been fulfilling.

(Vern)

Fine. I can be sexually attracted to adult males.

(Ethan)

I have had sex with adults (my ex-wife mainly)…Sex with my wife was usually good, often very good. I almost always fantasised that she was a child, and she often helped me by dressing as a schoolgirl. Sex with my wife was most satisfying when I successfully fantasised about her being a child.

(Lenny)

I'm really lucky, as while my preference is for girls aged eight to thirteen years old, I am also sexually attracted to adult women. I am therefore fine with the idea of sex with adults, and can have a perfectly satisfying sex life with a woman.

(Bill)

Answers such as Bill's, in which he says he 'can have a perfectly satisfying sex life with a woman', beg the obvious question of why, in that case, would someone continue to self-define as paedophile. My naïve expectation was that, if a person could be sexually attracted to adults, then any sexual attraction to children would diminish in significance and would become unimportant in their sense of self. Clearly, this is not how sexuality is experienced and the painful desperation shown in David's account (given in Chapter 1), where he is driven close to suicide by his attraction to boys even though he is also sexually attracted to women, provides a graphic example of how compelling the sexual attraction to children can feel even where it comprises only one component of one's total sexuality. The answers from these respondents provide a sense of a continuum in which sexual attraction to adults may form a more or less significant part of the total sexuality of individuals who remain committed to the self-definition of paedophile.

A small number of respondents talked about the wider significance of their relationships with adults, emphasising the aspect of deceit which they felt was inherent:

> *I **can** do it, but there is no passion in the act. … It left me feeling like I was unintentionally leading the other person on, into believing something very deep and personal was happening, and that this might lead to other things in the future (marriage, children, and so on). I also knew it to be ill-advised, to be having sexual relations 'just because'…or as a disguise.*
>
> (Steve)

> *I once had a sexual relationship with an adult woman so everyone would think I was normal, and it was not satisfying. I had to force myself to have sex with her.*
>
> (Justin)

> *I don't have any problem talking to or having sexual relations with women, the problem lies in long-term commitment. I think a marriage must be based on trust and honest communication and I do not think any woman – if she knew what I had – would want to be with me, and I'm not going to tell anyone to find out. It's a rock and a hard place but then, if I'm not willing to trust my life with someone then why should I expect her to trust her life with me? I have the odd one-night stand or short-term relationship but as such I don't have much of a drive to meet women and I blame 'A good heart these days is hard to find' or 'I work too much' and so on, to console friends who occasionally worry about this.*
>
> (John)

It is interesting to note that in this sample, where the question was answered, there appears to be roughly an even mix from negative, neutral and positive responses to the thought of having sex with adults. As discussed above, this finding challenged my own assumption that, if someone were able to have a satisfactory sexual relationship with an adult, then they would focus on that aspect of their sexual attraction. It makes clear that many paedophiles are not exclusively sexually attracted to under-age minors and yet their felt sexual attraction to children is regarded as highly significant and typically remains a defining part of the individual's identity – and often the biggest problem.

*I would say that being a ped consistently ranks as my biggest problem. I don't consider it a problem in the sense that simply having this attraction is problematic, instead what to **do** with it becomes the problem. ... I consider [being a paedophile] to be the biggest part of my identity.*

(Ben)

I do not personally regard this as 'my sexuality'. From a certain point of view it's kind of like when an anti-virus programme finds a suspicious file it can't delete and acts by moving it into a 'virus vault' or what I call fantasy. The computer technically still has the virus but it's just its ability to interact with the rest of the system is disabled. ... I prefer to work things out for myself.

(John)

Section II: Sources which shaped respondents' views of themselves

As respondents slowly and often painfully came to the realisation that they were different from those around them, they looked for further information, for role models and for images of paedophiles which they could relate to. I asked, 'What books, films, people, websites and so on have been important to you in shaping your view of yourself as someone sexually attracted to children?' Responses tended to be fairly complex and detailed, with respondents often mentioning a range of sources.

A minority of respondents emphasised that they had mainly relied on their own inner resources to develop their view of themselves, in the absence of positive information and indeed in the presence of negative information:

I must say that I don't relate nor need exterior things to shape my view of myself, I just look in my inner self for that.

(Carl)

I think my view of myself as a boylover was shaped long before I read a book on the subject, or saw a movie or website.

(Jerry)

Most importantly I feel that I, myself, have been important is shaping my view as someone sexually attracted to children.

(Stewart)

The persecution suffered undoubtedly shapes the view one has of oneself.

(Ethan)

When I hear about people being involved with children sexually it kind of sparks an interest when reading an article in the newspaper.

(Ian)

I am not very influenced by the views and perceptions of paedophilia in books, films and so on because they so often get it wrong. I suppose the book everyone thinks of is Lolita. *I love that novel as a piece of literary art, and Nabokov was such a great writer. But Humbert isn't exactly a character I relate to! Neither is* Lolita, *come to that.*

(William)

In the absence of good/honest information, many of my ideas about paedophilia have come from my own ideas and observations; and, of course, the little girls themselves have inspired many of my thoughts and feelings.

(Gary)

Other respondents wrote about specific websites, individuals or organisations which had helped them in developing a positive view of themselves:

These websites have helped me to understand my attractions to a greater extent, and to understand my place as a MAA in modern society.

(Ed, aged seventeen)

[A now-defunct website] where I developed my ethics as a BLer through contact with other people's experiences. I got to a new level of my sexual identity when I started to have a more distanced look on it, through scholar or semi-scholar works such as the Rind report.

(Bobby)

[A particular poster] whose experiences made him a hero to me, though I have never encountered him in real life. ... When I first acknowledged myself as a boylover, I spent a good deal of time on the web looking for stories and commentary and opinion to help me survey the territory: 'where does my internal life lie in the general map of human sexual fantasy?' The most important single component that these sites contributed to my general well-being was the personal stories of others. Not all personal tales are equally vivid or well-written – but most are emotionally instructive. I have benefitted beyond measure from the sum total of personal stories I've encountered on the web. ... The general level of moral candour and personal honesty, from the best threads and best posters to these groups, is breath-taking. It is intrinsically healthy and energising.

(Frank)

[A website] – this is the one and only constant that has educated me, and made me realise that I am not alone, I am not a freak, and I am not evil.

(Lenny)

Wikipedia helped me discover that there were people who believed that attraction to children was not evil, and that the predatory paedophiles in popular culture were not necessarily accurate depictions. [A now-defunct website] taught me a lot about who these people are.

(Kristof)

Nambla saved my life.

(Quentin)

[One site] made me consider paedophilia differently. Then [another site] made me understand who I really am and made me meet other boylovers.

(Raymond)

[Websites] have certainly helped me crystallise my identity as an MAA. ... My thinking has been changed by reading articles and research relating to paedophilia, and links to many of these have been discovered online. Also, I have clarified my own attitudes to many things, such as sexual activity with children, child pornography and so on, through discovering what other MAAs think about these issues. ... [A now-defunct website] was the first place I ever communicated with another MAA. It was quite a significant step at the time, and helped me a lot in dealing with real life issues.

(Tim)

The most important individuals to helping me accept my sexuality and move on with my life past the depression stage were other paedophiles I originally met online and then in person.

(Gus)

[A website] was the first BL board I encountered and the people on it have taught me that acceptance of yourself is the key to a stable personality. ... now I've accepted myself fully.

(Dirk)

What made me turn positively to sexuality was a book on Spartans. Reading on their home life showed an environment of homosexuality and pederasty. As one Spartan said, you are not a man until you have a boy in your bed.

(Marc)

As a teen in the 1940s, my father had an issue of Kinsey's Sexual Behaviour in the Human Male. *I referred to it often and wondered about myself while maturing. I still own the book.*

(Alan)

While many different books, individuals and so on were mentioned, a few recurred and seemed more significant than others. These included Nabokov's

Lolita (eight references), Tom O'Carroll's *Paedophilia: The Radical Case* (seven references), books by Edward Brongersma (five references) and Theo Sandfort (three references), the Kinsey *Reports* (three references), Judith Levine's *Harmful to Minors* (three references) and works by Frits Bernard, Fred Berlin, Magnus Hirschfield, John Money, Bruce Rind, Wilhelm Reich and 'sexologists' in general. James Kincaid's *Erotic Innocence* (1998) was also mentioned, and the American journalist Debbie Nathan. The most-cited literary authors were Lewis Carroll (Charles Dodgson) with six references, T. H. White (three references) and Mark Twain (Samuel Clemens) with two references, with references also to John Ruskin, Edgar Allen Poe, W. H. Auden, J. D. Salinger, William Mayne (a British children's author) and Joseph Geraci. Two books specifically on children's sexuality were cited, *Children and Sexuality* by Stevi Jackson and Will McBride's well-known sex-education book *Show Me.* Tony Duvert's *Good Sex Illustrated* was described by one respondent, Raymond, in the following terms: 'This book is an essay written by a French paedophile who defends the rights of children, including the right to make love.' Photographers Sally Mann and Jock Sturges, both of whom are well-known for nude portraits of children, were also mentioned as influential. Literary books and films cited by the respondents included, as well as the book and the two film versions of *Lolita* (which garnered eight references), *For a Lost Soldier* (five references), *Long Island Expressway, Lawn Dogs* and *Leon/The Professional* (each with four references), *Ponette* and *The Woodsman* (each with two references). Another significant film dealing with an explicitly paedophile theme, *Mysterious Skin,* was, perhaps surprisingly, referred to only once, while other works cited were *Dreamchild, The Man without a Face, Angela, Man on Fire,* and *Finding Neverland.* One seventeen-year-old respondent, Ulf, to the question 'What books, films, people, websites and so on have been important to you in shaping your view of yourself as someone sexually attracted to children?' noted of the book *Lolita* that it 'showed me what a bad child lover is like. But, it also really described how it feels to love children.' He also commented, '*The Professional* [*Leon*], obviously. Heart touching, and shows that children also are attracted to men in cases, and are able to make decisions.'

None of these works are particularly cheerful, and most have a grim if not bloody ending. For example, the plot of *For a Lost Soldier* (*Vor een verloren Soldaat,* dir. Roeland Koerbusch, 1992) involves a boy falling in love with a soldier who does not seem very emotionally warm towards the boy and who leaves without saying goodbye. *Long Island Expressway,* which is also known, tellingly, as *L.I.E.* (dir. Michael Cuesta, 2001) shows most adults as emotionally stunted and the paedophile character, by contrast, as more able to meet emotional needs – before he is murdered by a rejected former lover. *Dreamchild* (dir. Gavin Millar, 1985) is about the relationship between Lewis Carroll (Charles Dodgson) and his young friend Alice Liddell, and similarly *Finding Neverland* (dir. Marc Forster, 2004) explores the relationship between the playwright and author James Matthew Barrie and the four young boys of widow Sylvia Llewelyn Davies, a friendship which resulted in the acclaimed play and children's book *Peter Pan*. Grief and resilience are the subject of *Ponette* (dir. Jacques Doillon, 1996), which is about a four-year-old child coming to terms with the death of her mother, while *Angela* (dir. Rebecca Miller, 1995) explores madness and religious obsession and *The Man without a Face* (dir. Mel Gibson, 1993) is about the friendship between two troubled people, a young boy and a man with a disfigured face.

Lawn Dogs (dir. John Duigan, 1997), *Man on Fire* (dir. Tony Scott, 2004) and *Leon* (also known as *The Professional;* dir. Luc Besson, 1994) both show a gentle and complex relationship between an adult man and a young girl, where the child's emerging sexuality is only subtly acknowledged (and, in *Leon* and *Man on Fire,* is set against extreme and sustained violence and gunfire), while *The Woodsman* (dir. Nicole Kassell, 2004) and *Mysterious Skin* (dir. Greg Araki, 2004) both address the question of paedophilia head on. Of the two, *Mysterious Skin* is more graphic, echoing *L.I.E*'s portrayal of a young male prostitute but including a rape scene. Its focus is on how two young men cope with sexual abuse and it concludes on a tentatively optimistic note. *The Woodsman,* also, is permeated by ambiguity. Kevin Bacon plays a man sexually attracted to young girls; as the film progresses we are led to hope that he may be able to sustain an identity as the fairytale 'Woodsman' who can rescue Little Red Riding Hood (exemplified in the young girl Robin) in the woods from the Wolf of his own paedophile desires. It is a disturbing but ultimately hopeful tale. The challenging and sensitive portrayal of a paedophile in *The Woodsman* even prompted a post on one review site, the IMDb (Internet Movie Database), from someone who said 'Being myself a pedophile (I never intended to have sex with a child and I never will but I feel attraction pretty clearly) for the first time I found a movie that tryes [sic] to look at the pedophile from this point of view, to get in his head and to understand his feelings like a human being' ('Taleyran' 2008). However, it is clear that none of these films glamorises or condones paedophilia, although perhaps the two which arguably come closest in their sympathy for the central adult character and their invitation to the audience to share in the sexualisation of the child (*Lolita* and *Leon*) are also the most mainstream and the most commercial. My observation on this commercialisation of paedophile themes is by no means unique. Marianne Sinclair published *Hollywood Lolitas: The Nymphet Syndrome in the Movies* back in 1988, showing how Hollywood draws on paedophilic themes, and Kincaid (1998: 115), discussing the Shirley Temple phenomenon and her modern equivalents, provides a fascinating quote from the reporter Matthew Stadler. Stadler infiltrated a NAMBLA meeting and discovered that their 'secret eroticism' was simply network television, the Disney channel and mainline films: 'I had found NAMBLA's "porn", and it was Hollywood.'

Individuals named by respondents as being influential included the paedophile activists Lindsay Ashford (with eight references) and Kevin Brown, Tom O'Carroll and Jack McClellan (each with two references). At least four individuals known to have been involved in this research were cited by other respondents as having been influential to them. As well as individuals who have been at pains to portray paedophilia positively, it was interesting to note that respondents also included John Geoghan (a American Catholic priest sentenced for multiple sexual abuse of children and murdered while in prison), and the books *The Man They Called a Monster* (Wilson 1983) and *From Abused to Abuser* (Riegel 2005). Together with the comments by the respondents, it seems that, when individuals are searching for cultural contexts and role models by which to understand their own sexuality, they currently make use of negative role models (known sex offenders, newspaper items on sex offences, sexualised portrayals of children) as well as potentially more helpful models.

Section III: The significance of websites

One highly important source of information and models is undoubtedly websites. For the main questionnaire, respondents were asked to rate the main websites they visited in terms of 'how important this site has been to you' and to give details on how often they visited the sites and what contributions they made (posting articles, comments and so forth). Of the fifty-one respondents who provided this information, twelve listed one site as being of the greatest significance to them, twelve listed two sites and fourteen listed three main sites. The remaining thirteen listed four or multiple sites as being significant. As well as websites, respondents mentioned Internet chat (IRC) and Internet messaging (IM), email, mailing lists, private boards and also a radio station and podcast, but these seemed to most respondents in this sample to be less significant generally than visiting the public-access websites.

Around twenty-five current sites were listed in total, and around eight sites (such as Fresh Petals, Butterfly Kisses, Puellula, Talitha Koomi and Open Hands) believed to be defunct at present. (For a discussion of Puellula, see Goode 2008a.) Some sites change their names, and others (for example, Inquisition21, Tegenwicht and Freespirits) relate to libertarian ideas generally rather than specifically to paedophilia. Of those which are specifically aimed at the online paedophile community, two in particular stand out. These are the Internet forums for, respectively 'girl-lovers' and 'boy-lovers'. It may be partly an artefact of the sampling method that these two sites in particular (and their related offshoots) appear so significant, since the research project was advertised and discussed on these sites and thus would have attracted a higher proportion of regular site-visitors to participate in the study: on the other hand, the sites were chosen to advertise the project specifically because of their already-existing central importance to the online paedophile community.

As an example of where individuals sexually attracted to children may find their information, Bill, aged in his thirties, refers to Tom O'Carroll's *Paedophilia: The Radical Case* and a pamphlet made and distributed by CLogo, a 'girl-lover' website. Bill also lists Tom O'Carroll, Lindsay Ashford and Jack McClellan as important to him in shaping his view of himself, as well as listing six websites, including two – Absolute Zero and Perverted Justice – which are 'anti-paedophile' websites.

The major 'girl-lover' site was visited at least daily by fourteen of the respondents, and was rated as between 'eight' and 'ten' (highly important to the individual) by fourteen respondents. Sixteen of the respondents posted on this site at least occasionally. The equivalent 'boy-lover' site was visited at least several times a week by eleven of the respondents (although fewer posted on this site) and was rated as between 'eight' and 'ten' in importance by eight respondents. In total, there were forty-five instances of respondents visiting various paedophile sites on a 'frequent' basis (ranging from more than once a day to several times a week) and thirty-nine instances of sites rated as being important (with a rating of eight to ten). The contributions made by respondents to such sites ranged from being the web-editor or administrator to writing essays, articles, reviews, starting discussion threads, making comments and responses, messages and posting links. The nature of the contributions ran the gamut from humour, opinions, personal experiences and revelations, questions, factual replies, support and general chat. A check of such sites shows that much time can be devoted to posts about 'girlmoments' (known as GMs) and their equivalent 'boymoments'; in other words telling other posters about having seen (often from a distance, without any direct interaction) an attractive child. These anecdotes may be real or may be fictionalised mildly erotic, gloating or wistful stories. Time is also devoted to discussing particular child models or child actors, and films, Youtube videos or other places where children may be viewed. Posters also discuss going to foreign countries, and share information on legislation, as well as drawing attention to topical items in the news. On these publicly accessible and carefully moderated sites there is very little if any discussion of explicitly sexual topics. Rather, the chat is about relationships (actual or desired) with child 'friends' and especially about looking at and thinking about children and child-focused issues. There is a sense of building up a entire lifestyle centred on attraction to children, much as another individual might build up a lifestyle centred on being, for example, a 'Trekkie', a druid, a radio-ham or a Michael Jackson fan, with the main difference being that attraction to children is more likely to be kept hidden as a lifestyle. As one insider remarked in an email to me, 'A recurrent topic of discussion in-community is how much "culture" can one maintain in their home, without arousing suspicion; perhaps one can own all of Shirley Temple's movies, but shouldn't have any other child-themed movies so that a love of Shirley has plausible deniability.'

Posters also express their own sense of frustration, isolation, longing and rage, sometimes by extremely hostile remarks about adults who act protectively towards children, for example in an angry post about a mother (described as a 'shit-headed bitch') who stopped her young daughter from spending time with one of the posters.

The same names appear again and again on these sites and the constant chat on the same few repetitive topics builds up a sense of an established community with clear rules and conventions on how to behave. Visitors quickly learn which comments and questions will be welcomed and which may be ignored, trivialised or rebuked. As with any fan site or special-interest group – whether it be to do with celebrities, football teams, cars, sport, war-gaming, fantasy, porn or any other specialised (and predominantly masculine) interest – there is the focus on particular bodies of knowledge, specialised terminology, obsessive detail, and the one-upmanship of being more knowl-edgeable or more experienced than the rest. There is a shared sense of a spe-cial world, inaccessible to others, containing a unique and arcane knowledge. In this world, 'girl-love' or 'boy-love' is a precious gift, an exquisite aesthetic burden, a secret joy entrusted to the chosen few, which only those others within the community can truly understand and share. This seductive sense of solidarity with the community may be particularly valued in a context where one feels not only misunderstood but actively hated and despised by wider society. Thus the online community – drawing on the wider cultural resources such as the books, films, individuals and websites discussed earlier – can set up powerful shared understandings of what it means to be a 'paedophile' and how one may be expected to think, to feel and to behave. Part of the mechanism for encouraging conformity within this community certainly lies in the ways in which support is offered to its members and this is discussed in Chapter 8, but before looking at the question of support we will turn our attention to another aspect of respondents' interior lives, their fantasies.

7　Attraction and fantasies

I suppose you just can't keep getting shocked at the same thing time and again.

(John)

Introduction

Before moving on to explore their interactions with others within and outside
the online paedophile community, it is worth looking at what respondents
wrote about another aspect of their interior life – their fantasies. In this
chapter, two main aspects are examined. The first of these concerns the
'triggers' in the external world which the respondents experienced as sexually
attractive. In the main questionnaire, I asked (after asking what age-range
respondents found attractive) 'What is it about this age group that most
attracts you?' My aim was to try to tease out the perceived aspects of physical
attractiveness (smooth skin and so on) from the perceived aspects of psychological attractiveness (open, trusting and suchlike qualities). There were also
aspects of social attributes, such as playfulness and curiosity, which are
shared with adults but which are more likely to be encouraged or accepted
in children.

Alongside these aspects of real children, I wanted to know about the idealised
children in respondents' minds, and the scenarios which they played out in
fantasy. The questions I asked in the main questionnaire were 'Do you have
fantasies concerning relationships with children? If so, how often? What happens in these fantasies? When you have these fantasies, how do you respond?
What do you do?' The rationale behind this flurry of rather probing questions
was to try to find out (without asking incriminating questions) the ways in
which individuals might link their sexual fantasy with action in the real
world. Some respondents waxed extremely lyrical on these subjects and literally wrote pages. Others were more curt, giving answers of just a few words.
Given the context of a written questionnaire, which can appear quite cold and
clinical as well as intrusive, I was not surprised that some respondents
declined to go into any details. I was all the more pleased, therefore, that
some respondents made such an effort to explain their inner lives.

In this chapter, therefore, Section I explores the question of children's attractiveness to the respondents and Section II provides quotations on the range of sexual and romantic fantasies provided by the respondents.

Section I: 'What is it about this age group that most attracts you?'

On the subject of attractiveness, only one, Raymond, commented, 'I am not attracted by children in general, but by individuals', and John wrote 'Just a feeling'. Two others, Adrian and Xavier, did not answer this question. The remaining forty-six respondents gave informative and often detailed answers.

Twenty-eight of the forty-six respondents made reference to physical attributes, including features of 'natural beauty', size, proportion, smooth skin, softness and hairlessness. Several waxed lyrical about the 'stunning beauty' of the child's 'perfect body' (Patrice), with Louis commenting 'I find the sight of them overwhelmingly glorious' and William and Tim both writing over two pages on features they find attractive. Only one respondent, Ian, referred explicitly to 'undeveloped genitals', while for Eustace it is the girl's giggle which is most significant and for Hugo and Kristof the sound of the child's voice. Seven respondents spoke about the 'magical time' of being 'right on the brink of puberty' (Jerry), a 'process of flowering open' (Dirk) and an 'intermediate', 'limbo' or liminal stage as the child moves from pre-puberty into puberty and hence into adulthood. Only Ken spoke about this stage in terms of a girl 'becoming sexually aware', while for others such as Tim this moment seemed more spiritual in significance.

Tim was the only respondent to refer to the technical description of the 'Tanner stages', a system used to classify stages of puberty and one which deserves a brief excursus. The system of Tanner stages was developed in 1969 as a result of a twenty-year study (the Harpenden Growth Study) by a research team led by a British paediatrician, Dr James Mourilyan Tanner (born 1920), under the auspices of the Institute of Child Health at the University of London. Tanner and his team chose to perform this longitudinal study (which focused on detailed study and photography of the breasts and pubic areas, every three months, of children aged from perhaps six or seven years old up to around fifteen or sixteen years old) by using children who were living in children's homes (Hall 2006: 63). There is no mention in the published reports (Marshall and Tanner 1969, 1970) of any ethics procedures or protocols of informed consent followed during this study. Under 'Material and Methods', the authors state of their subjects (192 girls and 228 boys) that they

> lived in family groups in a children's home where the standard of care was in all respects excellent. They came mainly from the lower socio-economic sector of the population, and some may not have received optimal physical care before entering the home (usually between age 3 and 6 years). The reason for their admission was usually break-up of the parental home by divorce or by death, illness, or desertion of one parent.
>
> (Marshal and Tanner 1969: 291)

In other words, these were typically the children of impoverished single mothers (but described as 'orphans'): the researchers had apparently chosen a sample of highly vulnerable children, with disempowered parents, who could presumably more easily be coerced into complying with these intrusive examinations. To do the study, Tanner took on an assistant, Reginald White-house, who was '[i]nnocent of any academic training' but had been in the Army, a 'robust man', with a 'peremptory, no-nonsense bearing' who could keep 'squirming, recalcitrant children under control' (Hall 2006: 62–3). The results of this study were published in reputable medical journals and thus data which seem to have been obtained by bullying extremely vulnerable children into repeatedly being photographed and measured in a highly intrusive manner are now regarded as classic texts which have been used by clinicians ever since.

Six of the respondents referred to 'cuteness', which is an attribute which seems to fall somewhere between physical appearance and psychological mannerisms, and two respondents (Victor and Max) simply answered 'personality' as being attractive, but other respondents said a great deal about the psychological characteristics, writing about the following qualities:

Free-spirited, spontaneous.

(Ben)

Natural curiosity and wonder, quality of not being beat down by the world.

(Gary)

Natural, uninhibited, unprejudiced, keen to learn.

(Nigel)

Outgoing, imaginative, think for themselves.

(Anne)

Spontaneity, vitality.

(Pete)

Playful yet reserved personality, unbiased perspective to people in general.
(Ralph)

Attitude, openness, joy, happiness.

(Stewart)

Not being influenced by common opinions or standards.

(Vern)

Excitement for life, lack of disillusionment, enjoyment of simple things.
(Bernice)

Open-mindedness, sense of life's potential, not yet indoctrinated by society.

(Ethan)

Sincerity.

(Freddy, aged sixteen)

Open-mindedness towards life.

(Gavin)

Values, views on things.

(Hugo)

The way they act.

(Kristof)

Curiosity, playfulness, vulnerability, gentleness, energy, exuberance.

(Louis)

Fresh outlook on life, playfulness.

(Marc)

Brains developed for independent thinking, without being conditioned to conform.

(Andy)

Typical behaviour of boys, honest, free, discovering, experiencing, wide-minded, brave.

(Oscar)

Joy of life.

(Patrice)

Neville commented that children are 'wonderful people to have a conversation with', and Todd found attractive 'how they react to the attention I give them, usually very positively', while Ulf (aged sixteen) summed it up as 'everything, souls, bodies, minds…how they feel in my arms – to simply hold them, and nothing else. How everything is so magical and special to them'. Only Ian (who had also referred to 'undeveloped genitals' and who later emailed me claiming to have raped a child) specifically mentioned the quality of 'innocence' as attractive. Four respondents mentioned sexual aspects explicitly:

High sex drive, adventurous.

(Wayne)

Natural eroticness, explorative, playful.

(Steve)

Sexually desirable, utterly joyous, bursting with enthusiasm.

(Thomas)

Spontaneity, happiness, sense of love. Sex is just a small part of the whole equation. I can't think of anything I would like to do more than simply spend some time in their company.

(Bill)

For Louis, the attraction included fatherly elements: he commented that he felt 'Paternal. I have a strong desire to be a good influence in their lives'.

Thus, for the forty-six people in this group, there were twenty-eight references to physical attributes and twenty-nine to non-physical (psychological or social) attributes, with the non-physical attributes being described in greater detail. For a small number of respondents, such as John, the attraction to children seems to be incidental, unwanted, to be firmly put to one side whenever possible. For others, attraction to children is something to revel in and is presented as the basis for an entire identity and lifestyle. The following edited extracts draw out the major themes identified by William and Tim, who contributed over two pages of answers each.

*To me, there is simply nothing on this earth as beautiful...subtlety and understated spiritual power. ... the incredible power she has to affect and move me, to bring me to my knees in awe and adoration!...The superlatives are not superlative enough. ... Lewis Carroll in one of his letters, wrote of experiencing a 'feeling of reverence, as at the presence of something sacred' when he was photographing certain of his child friends 'undraped'. ... sensitivity...an awareness of and interest in other people and other living things; care and compassion; gentleness. ... [After my mother died] a Little Girl...as she was sat reading to me, she took my hand into hers and gently stroked it; her expression showed that she knew I was hurting (the children had been told) and she badly wanted to comfort me. I can vividly recall the feeling of a power surge: life and feeling returning to me and enlivening me again. ... Beauty of spirit clothed in the beauty of form. ... playfulness...wonderfully infectious and lively wit, eccentricity and charm...gentle 'teasing' which is really about a Little Girl knowing that you like her, and her delight in that, testing it out, enjoying your responses to her...And, probably, most people – or most decent people anyway – would agree up to a certain point: little girls **are** beautiful, cute and charming. So how is this 'paedophilic'? How is it sexual? Well, the point is that the beauty and loveliness of little girls, which I have tried my best – inevitably rather inadequately – to describe above, is to me utterly **sexy**. It* *is erotically appealing. ... I am moved **romantically**. ... Girl Love is, to me, a 'sexuality – plus'. If that makes sense! It is **everything** to me, the core of my identity as a person, and everything that is most significant and important to me.*

(William)

Secret, sensual, intensely imaginative, passionate, curious. ... Their love of glitter and pink and magic wands and fairy wings is a celebration of paganism and extravagance. ... Kneeling in the garden mixing up a magic potion of flower petals and water, my feelings are that I am beside a fountain of creativity, and that whatever threadbare image or faded narrative I drop into it will emerge coloured like a Disney feature and glistening with life...The bloom of youth, liminal stage. ... It's clear to me in hindsight that as I went through puberty I grew increasingly nostalgic for girls as equals, with the physical confidence they had as pre-adolescents.

(Tim)

I have not made a distinction in this analysis between those respondents who are primarily attracted to girls, boys or both, or those who are attracted to those children at the younger or older ends of the age-spectrum. Instead, what seems to be conveyed by this small sample of forty-six individuals writing about what they find most attractive in children is the sense of children as whole people, albeit highly idealised. This sample of individuals do not, in general, seem to be focusing on or fetishising certain body parts, as many heterosexual men do with adult women's breasts, buttocks or legs, or as many homosexual men do with body-hair or musculature. If anything, what is being fetishised in these responses is not physical attributes but a particular moment of uncomplicated joyousness and freedom. It seems that what is desired here (as well as sexual contact with a child) is contact with a moment in life before adult restraints and conformities press down. The adult desires the playfulness, curiosity, open-mindedness, energy, excitement and pleasure which children are seen to embody.

For many adults, leaving childhood behind and entering on the path to adulthood has meant losses as well as gains. I can distinctly remember that, as a child, there was little in adulthood, and especially in womanhood, which seemed attractive in prospect. I took pleasure in my small narrow body which could squeeze through railings and thus liberate me out into the woodlands. I relished being able to take off my top on hot summer days and resented the thought of having to cover up. I loved being able to slip unnoticed among people, without the stares and ogles of adolescent boys. As I grew older, I felt my body changing against my will and beyond my control, clumsy and large, aching with period pains, sweating and smelling. All the benefits of childhood – the immediacy of friendship, the comfortable and easy hand-holding and sharing of secrets, the intense imaginative life in which one can spend entire hours or even days immersed in one's own created world, un-selfconsciously talking to oneself, utterly caught up in the concentration of the moment – all this becomes laughable, and derisory, as the years pass and the threshold of puberty is reached. For girls, what is lost is too often that sense of bodily autonomy, that 'physical confidence' that Tim describes, as the emerging woman become the sexualised and constrained object of male gaze. For boys, what is lost is more likely to be their untroubled access to a rich emotional life and to the background comfort of friendly touch; the hugs, hand-holding and affectionate kisses of early boyhood. Ironically, then, what is being idealised and desired by paedophiles are exactly those child-like qualities which adults typically collude in socialising out of children.

Section II: Romantic and sexual fantasies

Finding oneself sexually attracted often leads to fantasies about desired scenarios. Only one respondent, aged in his seventies, stated that he did not fantasise, and one 'preferred not to say'. Eustace made the point that there are a number of aspects to fantasy, which

> [c]ould be about a strong desire for something to happen and trying to make it happen, or wishing something would happen while knowing it won't, or just imagining something while not caring whether it ever happens or not, or imagining something while wanting it to **not** happen. People of all types have 'fantasies' about things they want and try to get, and about things they just enjoy imagining that they know they'll never have, and things they imagine that they don't want to come true.

This conflation of the different meanings of 'fantasy', including planning, desiring, hoping, wishing or dreaming, with both longing and ambivalence, are evident to some extent in the answers of these respondents.

Of the forty-eight respondents who gave information about their fantasies, eighteen described having fantasies about children 'all the time' (Max), more than once a day (Ian, Bobby, William, Dirk), daily (ten respondents), or 'almost everyday' (Carl, Bill, Hans). A further thirteen described fantasising 'frequently', 'most days' or 'several times a week', with a further three fantasising weekly. Vern described fantasising 'not too rarely' and Derek and Andy 'relatively rarely'. The remaining eleven respondents did not quantify how often they fantasised. Therefore, of the thirty-seven respondents who gave information on how often they fantasised about children, thirty-one of the thirty-seven fantasised at least weekly, with fifteen of these fantasising at least daily. Around twenty-three of the respondents wrote that they responded to the fantasy by masturbating. Thus fantasy appears to play a significant role in the lives of these individuals, a role which is repeatedly reinforced by masturbation on at least a weekly basis for the majority. What was it they fantasised about? Fantasies contained a number of different elements or aspects and therefore do not lend themselves to easy analysis and categorisation.

However, there are a number of distinguishing features which can be identified in this sample of forty-eight fantasies.

In this sample, no respondent referred directly to non-consensual or aggressive sexual activity, although three respondents gave accounts of fantasies which appeared purely sexual with no obvious component of affection or relationship. Vern fantasised about 'Introducing sexual acts, evolves into a long chain usually lasting more than two months, continuously developing the story further from the point I last left it alone. I respond by arousal and masturbation', and the other two respondents wrote about exclusively sexual fantasies which appeared to be potentially harsh: Lenny (who has two convictions for accessing child pornography) has been fantasising for over thirty years, weekly, using the imagery of directing a porn movie in which numerous men 'do things' to passive 'innocent' little girls, culminating in an image of 'numerous ejaculating men', leaving Lenny 'with a euphoric feeling and a sense of well-being'. Ian, who is sexually attracted to babies, who talks about being sexually 'addicted' to small children and who claims to act on his attractions is, in my view, the most disturbing of the respondents: 'all my fantasies that I have include sexual relations with young children [from infancy upwards]. I have these fantasies about two or three times a day. In the fantasies I am either having sexual intercourse with the child or some type of oral or body rubbing activity with the child. I am often very sexually aroused when I am having these fantasies and always masturbating to these thoughts.'

Other fantasies, while still predominantly sexual, referred to elements such as kissing, cuddling and mutuality. Steve fantasises several times a month: 'Normally, I am caressing, kissing and explore a child's naked body. This leads into masturbating the child, and performing oral sex on him. I become very highly aroused, and normally masturbate to the most amazingly intense orgasm. Or write down fantasies in an erotic story.' Quentin fantasises 'several times a week' about 'mutual masturbation or mutual oral sex. I masturbate and then go about my daily business.' Ralph fantasises about 'play, talking, kissing, holding hands, to masturbation and dry-intercourse. Masturbate or redirect my focus to daily tasks.' Hans, 'daily to every few days', fantasises about 'being with a loved boy, holding him, cuddling with him. In some cases, I fantasise touching or performing oral sex on him. Occasionally the fantasies lead to masturbation.' Clive fantasises 'several times a week' that 'we undress each other and engage in various activities up to and including intercourse, depending on the age of the child. Masturbate. I also write erotic stories.' Bernice similarly fantasises about 'fondling and caressing'. Nigel fantasises 'most days' about 'intimate contact (kissing, cuddling, fondling), sometimes leads to masturbation', and, for Marc, fantasy 'usually involves embracing (hugging, kissing). In the past used to be far more sexual content.' Kristof responded: 'I would classify them more as thoughts than fantasies, but they occur rather frequently. They typically involve hugging and cuddling, and sometimes light sexual interaction. Mostly the thoughts simply pass as my mind moves on to other things. Sometimes I masturbate.'

Thus, of the forty-eight fantasies given, twelve contained predominantly sexual imagery, of which three appeared exclusively sexual and nine involved some element of caressing within the sexual contact. Of the rest, around fourteen of the respondents brought in elements of 'platonic', 'romantic' or 'friendship-based' daydreams as well as explicitly sexual masturbation fantasies, with Ben stating: 'Sometimes totally sexual, sometimes totally platonic, sometimes in-between. Daydream about being with a little girl in one of these ways, and just enjoy the daydream.' Todd similarly reported on daily fantasies, 'The fantasies can be very sexual or sometimes I just see myself together with a young girl, enjoying her company', as did Ethan, who fantasised 'frequently', 'Sometimes sexual, sometimes not, spending time together, walking on a beach, watching a movie, laughing, having fun, talking. Don't try to push the fantasies away, just enjoy them and continue with life.' This sense of incorporating fantasies about children into everyday life came across in a number of responses. Victor's daily fantasies 'are about meeting someone, becoming close friends, cuddling and kissing' and Neville reported, 'Once a month or so I dream I am a parent of a little boy, five years old or so, and I am nice to him, treating him real well and he responds to me by kissing me on the lips.' Thomas exemplified both the distinction between non-sexual and sexual fantasy and also the incorporation of fantasy in daily life:

> *Daily. Two types. First type is more like a daydream where I imagine including little girls in my daily activities. I could be driving to the store, and I will imagine that a little girl was going with me, and imagine what we would talk about on the ride there. If I'm eating a meal alone, I sometimes imagine that I'm sharing that meal with a little girl, and imagine what we would talk about as we ate. The daydream fantasies are just part of my daily life. The second type would be sexual fantasies where I imagine engaging in sexual activities with little girls. I imagine a broad range of activities, from just cuddling with a little girl, to having intercourse with girls at the very upper end of my preferred age range (twelve years). None of my fantasies involve hurting little girls or doing anything against their wishes. I don't think there's anything inherently wrong with having fantasies of non-consensual sex, but the idea of hurting or forcing a little girl just doesn't arouse me, in fact, they have quite the opposite effect. The sexual fantasies are masturbation fantasies. Combined with legal pictures of little girls, the sexual fantasies are my only sexual outlet. My wife and I do not have sex. ... When I realise I'm getting aroused, I find a time and place to be alone and fantasise about little girls and masturbate.*

Like Thomas, other respondents also emphasised the 'consensual' or 'harmless' nature of their fantasies. Ken said of his daily fantasies that they are about 'touching them, rubbing up against them, licking them, kissing them, caressing them, masturbating, oral sex, it's all very gentle and consensual'. Carl also noted that he has fantasies 'almost everyday' which involve 'Nothing that hurts the child. I often masturbate.'

Four of the respondents appeared to fantasise mainly about children known to them in real life. Adrian fantasises daily about 'memories of past relationships'. Raymond focuses on one particular boy in real life: 'I mostly imagine myself making love with him. More particularly I imagine myself giving him pleasure, mostly by masturbation or fellation. In these fantasies the boy is always wanting; as I love this boy I could not possibly think of hurting him in any way possible. On the contrary I'd like to protect him and help him. And also give him pleasure, but only if he wants me to.' Stewart fantasises about children he has seen: 'Just yesterday I saw a girl in a public area around ten years old, all I could think about was ballroom dancing with her and she was wearing a lovely white gown. I usually just go about my regular day or back to whatever I'm doing. I don't really try to stop myself from having them, some of them are quite pleasant.' William expanded on his experiences:

Several times each day. I recall experiences with Little Girls from my real life – perfectly legal, non-sexual experiences – and then focus on these in fantasies; I 'eroticise' them mentally. I'm not sure what you mean by 'how do I respond'. I don't act them out in reality, if that is what you mean. I dwell upon them in fantasy, and often masturbate to them. Perhaps that would sound sordid to some people, but it isn't. I see fantasy as having a number of functions. First, it allows me to express myself sexually in the only legal way that I can do that; second, because of this, it acts as a release of sexual frustration and tension; third, it is sometimes quite a reflective experience: it allows me to reflect on my feelings. ... I want to try to get as close as I can to 'feeling' the Girl's feelings. ... I think beautiful Little Girls are just amazing, and I want to gain a sense of what it must feel like to be the Girl, and to be the Girl in the situation of being adored, being loved, being made love to.

Four respondents had fantasies about scenarios with themes of seduction or rescue. These scenarios are common in our culture, for example in Hollywood movies. As Kincaid, among others, has identified, such scenarios about pre-teen children are part of our standard shared cultural fantasies:

Current films work obsessively with a single plot: a child, most often a boy, possessed either of no father or a bad one, is isolated, sexualised, and imperilled, whereupon he or she runs into an adult, often a male, who is down on his or her luck, outcast, misunderstood, sensitive, on the lam, romantically irresistible – usually all of these, and always the last. The child falls in love, initiates the love, and it blossoms, fed eagerly by the child and resisted by the reluctant adult, who is, however, finally overcome as the love takes over, bigger than both of them.

(Kincaid 1998: 115)

Bobby related how he fantasises

> *every night, as a way to enter into sleep, imaginary casual relationships*
> *with boys (between two boys, between a boy and an adult, or between a*
> *boy and me) [which develops into] a story of seduction by the boy, and*
> *then (if I'm not asleep yet!) a sexual relationship. At that moment I may*
> *masturbate or not. I do also masturbate about once a day when I'm fully*
> *awake, then the scenarios are more directly sexual, with the help of photos*
> *or films. I daydream about boys too, but then the scenarios are not sexual.*

The two youngest respondents, Ulf and Freddy, both aged sixteen, have
fantasies about rescue. Freddy fantasises daily, explaining: 'I try to work my
paedophilic imaginations into longer "epic" fantasies, and the child is typically introduced as a character I must rescue (and eventually do). At some
point I will cuddle with her, and kiss. And sometimes I have spontaneous
fantasies which just skip to the snuggling part', while Ulf fantasises 'at least
twice a week' about a scenario

> *where I find a girl, hurt, alone in the woods, naked – defenceless, you name*
> *it. I immediately pick her up, and then take her to my home. My parents*
> *object as I place her in bed, and take care of her with warm clothing, good*
> *food, and try to at least give her medical support. Then there'll be the part*
> *where she starts crying, and I hold her for what seems hours. And, that's it.*

Similarly, Justin explained: 'Sometimes I fantasise about being the friend of
a misunderstood or lonely child. Usually happens when I am bored. The
fantasies bring some pleasure, but I try to tell myself when I have them that
they are merely a side effect of my sexual attraction to children.'

Section III: The relationship between fantasy and real life

At this point, it is relevant to try to link what was going on in respondents'
heads with what might be happening, or likely to happen, in real life. Around
20 per cent of the sample spontaneously made this explicit link. Thus, like
Justin quoted above, a further ten of the forty-eight respondents also made
careful distinctions between what is fantasy and what is reality, highlighting
that what occurred in fantasy would not take place in real life.

For example, Ben commented 'I don't act on my fantasies in real life.' Jerry
uses specific fantasies to make this clear in his own mind, describing how his
fantasy life is

> *rich and varied, in response, I suppose, to my not engaging in any real life*
> *sexual behaviour. Two basic types, either I'm in a relationship with a boy,*
> *or I myself am a boy in a relationship with other boys. ... the boy is usually*
> *not real in some fashion [robot, hologram]. [Because of having been*

arrested] I can't imagine putting another boy through the hell my young friend subsequently underwent. The non-human boys in my fantasies are my way of being able to love these boys, and be loved in return, even in my own imagination, without the possibility of harm coming to them.

Gary stated that he had been fantasising about children for over twenty years and that 'I alleviate my fantasies/desires through masturbation but I also channel my thoughts and feelings toward my art and my fiction. In other words, I seek healthy outlets that do not involve actual children in any direct way.' Max admitted that he fantasises 'all the time, but never act on them as it's a fantasy not real. What it would be like to see them naked and wonder if they would enjoy sexual experience. I sometimes masturbate to them but not always.' Pete similarly fantasises 'daily' about scenarios which are 'not always explicitly sexual. Friendship followed by bodily contact followed by sexual. Thinking: this is only fantasy – keep a sharp eye on the reality. Laying in bed, I might masturbate.' Gavin wrote about how fantasies 'pop in and out of my head regularly. But they remain just what they are: fantasies, and I don't go out to make them real. As to the content of these fantasies, they range from platonic relationships to sexually explicit ones.' Derek also realises his fantasies are

profoundly unrealistic, since I'm not good with children in real life. My fantasy child has properties such as being as intelligent and mature and sexually willing as an adult. I often picture myself in a subservient role. My fantasies are most likely to take the form of purely sexual play. ... I ignore it, masturbate, or sober up.

Oscar fantasises 'three to four times a week' about

having concrete sex with boys. I only have those fantasies during masturbation. If I see a handsome boy I sometimes fantasise about how he would look naked. It makes me horny. During masturbation I always try to focus on children I don't know (by way of pictures). This is because I don't want to feel strongly attracted and horny to children I actually know and meet. This is a way how I try to protect myself from abusing children.

Tim wrote that fantasising about children he knows in real life would make him feel 'creepy', explaining that he fantasises daily

almost exclusively about sexual interactions with children. There isn't much dialogue and the fantasies rarely involve children I know. I don't make an effort not to fantasise about child friends, I just don't seem to do it much. I guess it makes me feel creepy. I make the effort to fantasise about sex with adults sometimes, because I want to attenuate my sexual associations with kids if I can. Most of the time it just doesn't work for me... [fantasies] often involve me giving a child (typically a girl) oral sex. I seldom fantasise about penetrating a child, unless it's minimally with my tongue, and I seldom think of the child touching my penis or pleasuring me in any way. I'm always focused on giving the child pleasure. The ultimate sexual experience for me would be to give a little girl cunnilingus and make her come.

He wrote about his feelings of guilt, but 'guilt has never helped me control my urges though. Quite the opposite. It's only since I've fully accepted my sexual feelings, and examined them without judgement, that I've remotely considered ways to integrate them better with social norms.'

Louis gave a longer response which encompassed the 'self-control' technique of allowing himself to think about real-life boys while avoiding having sexual fantasies about them:

I'd love to marry a boy. I am only able to reach orgasm when fantasising about engaging sexually with a boy. … I have two kinds of fantasies about relationships with children. One I find acceptable and the other I tolerate as a means of self-control. In the first kind I fantasise spending time with kids in appropriate situations. Playing games, hugging, wrestling, singing, going on adventures – just hanging out and doing stuff together. These fantasies sometimes involve real boys in my life. I dream of calling them up and saying hi on the phone or tucking them into bed at night, or playing with them. Sometimes I'll relive a conversation we had in the real world or something we did together – that brings me so much joy often moving me to laughter or tears. Most often these fantasies involve made up boys or an imagined me as a boy. Often I imagine that I am a boy myself. I have fantasised like this since I was very young. During my teen and young adult years the fantasies would involve me being a super-hero and rescuing the boy from some evil bad-guy – now I'm happier just imagining a friendship. These fantasies I would have several times a day, every day, particularly when I'm on my own and not doing much else (e.g., when I'm driving). The second kind of fantasy involves sexing up a boy accompanied with masturbation. I am usually oral sexing him and he is always really enjoy- ing it. The idea of me pleasuring a boy is the motivation of these fantasies. I am careful to not use real boys that I know in these fantasies. I don't feel completely at ease with these fantasies – but if I don't have regular sexual release I find myself tempted to fantasise about real boys, to be more sexually interested in real boys, to follow boys around in shopping centres and public places and then I get dreams about sexing with said boys [the boys followed in real life] which I find most distressing. Because in my dreams I do things (e.g., force a boy to have sex or have sex with a boy I know) that I would not allow myself to fantasise about consciously. I find these fantasies and masturbation sessions very gratifying. Sexual fantasies will pop into my mind several times a day also, but usually I dismiss them. It is only a couple of times a week that I'll masturbate and really allow the fantasy.

While four of the respondents wrote casually about their sexual fantasies, remarking 'I'm not bothered' (Oliver) or 'I accept these fantasies as part of a normal polymorphous human sexuality' (Wayne), three respondents – in addition to Louis – mentioned having been distressed by their fantasies or the impossibility of acting on them. Bill, who fantasises almost every day about being submissive to a sexually active girl, commented:

> *When I first started having these fantasies as an adolescent they made me feel very guilty and ashamed, and I felt like a bad person because of them, but now I do not feel any guilt about them. As far as I am concerned, they do not harm anyone and I do not feel any reason to be ashamed of them anymore.*

Dirk, who fantasises at least daily, wrote: 'If I feel good I just dream and enjoy the fantasy. If I feel depressed I'm going to cry thinking about the near impossibility of acceptance. When I have such fantasies in bed I relieve myself of sexual tension.' Anne, similarly, wrote her fantasies were about 'Being in a world where society doesn't hate me and I can be in a relationship as I please. Romantic not sexual. I end up getting really mad at myself and sometimes I attempt suicide because I think the relationship will never happen.'

Patrice, on the other hand, seemed to be the only respondent who appeared to be planning to make his fantasy come true, writing that he often dreams

> *about finding a boy and having a true and loving relationship with him: I think this is a goal of many boylovers, similar to what Peyrefitte, Gide or Wilde experienced during their life. It's not about sex, it's really about love. The only possible response is to try your best to find this special boy and the only way to do that is to see boys often: camps, lessons, sports and so on.*

Two respondents, Xavier and John, wrote about how they managed their fantasies by simply allowing them to happen. Xavier wrote about how

> *I have a lot of wishful thinking. More than anything I would like to have an intimate (non sexual) relationship with a young girl. I think about this often. … Sexual fantasies…one to three times a week. Take place in the context of a consensual relationship, I imagine just holding her in my arms, and kissing her warm skin. I might venture lower, providing her oral sti-mulation, and inducing an orgasm. I find that highly erotic. I have learned to embrace my fantasies without encouraging them. In other words, I let them happen, but do not deliberately seek to have them. I do not deny them anymore either. I have found that when I sought to deny my thoughts they became intrusive over the course of my day to day life. Since I have allowed myself the freedom to fantasise about children I can honestly say my fantasies are not ever-present, as in they only occur during masturbation and rarely outside that.*

John wrote that he fantasises

[o]nce a day usually before I get out of bed. It lasts for no more than five minutes and that's more or less the last I think about it during the day. … I might have a fantasy before I go to sleep especially if I'm having trouble sleeping. … The basic fantasy is structured around me and a boy who are somehow friends, scented candles, massage oils and is more about sensuality and fun. The boy doesn't do anything to me and there is no anal sex…an extended fantasy which involves me helping my 'boy friend' with his maths homework and seeing a big smile from him when he gets an A in his exams or taking him out for a game of golf with a view to helping him be the next Tiger Woods. It generates in me a nice feeling of accomplishment to be a part of his success, I'm happy for him. … I do not fear it anymore and I suppose you just can't keep getting shocked at the same thing time and again. At this stage in my life I just leave it to do 'its thing'. It's just something odd about me. … I just give it some room and leave it at that.

Unusually, John stayed in touch with me throughout the analysis and writing up of the project, and took the opportunity to reflect further, commenting how the fantasies he had of helping young teenage boys were

the backdrop to a phenomenal and completely overwhelming feeling of failure and the deepest misery, hurt, isolation and fear that undermined the very value of my life itself…[When the boy] becomes the next Roy Keane then everyone else will say that my life and existence added to all that is positive and people would love me for it and I would be truly happy and have a purpose in this life. Since then I have worked my way out of that blind misery and have brought a real peace and understanding about myself and others. The qualities I admired in boys, I now feel I've rediscovered within myself. I've come to the realisation that the transition to adulthood was not to leave them behind. They were merely buried under so much fear, confusion and pain. I feel I've now won back my sense of wonder, curiosity, questioning, optimism about the future, kindness, compassion, playfulness and wanting to do plain old good!…It's been a couple of years now since I've had those 'extended fantasies' and I'm glad I will not be wasting any more time on them. … Why would I want a relationship with a twelve-year-old boy? It sounds so ridiculous now after winning back so much in terms of my family, friends and life. … I have had to validate and justify my own existence in a way perhaps others haven't. … [By] focusing more on what's really good for myself I have 'inadvertently' created a personal safe environment in which any child is as safe around me as they are around anyone else, now and in the future.

The process that John alludes to, in relation to rediscovering, reclaiming and reintegrating his own innate sense of boyishness into his mature adult self (together with a more conscious acknowledgement of his desire for achievement and appreciation of his own merits rather than vicariously), seems to point towards one very positive way of managing fantasies, making use of their psychic energy as a motor for personal growth.

Taking an overview of all the fantasies given by the respondents, what is interesting is their often gentle, yearning, nature. This is not what we might be led to expect from the current view of paedophiles as horrific, sadistic monsters. These fantasies are in fact a relief – having read them, perhaps we need be less afraid. They appear, in at least fourteen of the responses, to be about friendship as much as sexual contact, and in around thirteen of the responses there is an element of managing or controlling the fantasy, for example by the individual consciously reminding himself that this is not 'real life'. Four of the respondents (Louis, Justin, Ulf and Freddy) incorporated elements of being a rescuer or 'super-hero' into their fantasies (even though part of the 'rescue' might include eventual sexual contact with the child). There is of course the possibility that the respondents deliberately downplayed or censored their fantasies to make them more socially acceptable, and this may account for the absence of violent and coercive descriptions. Even with that proviso, however, these fantasies seem generally to reflect a genuine sanity and caring, an underlying desire to please and not to harm the child.

Although I wince at descriptions of cunnilingus or fellatio with children, I notice also the many references to cuddling, sharing and friendship and they give me hope. If we compare these fantasies with those of the sample of more than 3,000 men collected by the writer Nancy Friday in *Men in Love* (Friday 2003), which is perhaps the most comprehensive collection of male sexual fantasies published to date, we can see that what sets the paedophile respondents apart is often the greater emphasis on non-sexual friendship and doing 'everyday' things together such as sharing meals or walking on the beach. These are fantasies that may be plastic, that may be capable of being shaped over time into more (or less) socially acceptable forms. Friday makes the point in her books (for example, see Friday 1992), as her research on women's and men's fantasies has continued over decades, that fantasies change as the economic, political, social and cultural climate changes. Sexual fantasies are not only the private interior world of the individual: they are built out of the cultural material around us, including the pornography, the films, the books and the cultural feedback available to us. Thus, as a society, we have some responsibility for, and some control over, the fantasies which each of us secretly harbour. The fantasies described today may be very different from those twenty years ago – and from those twenty years from now. And, as Friday (along with many others) has observed, 'We must not confuse fantasy wishes with desires we hope will come true. Some people would like to act out their fantasies. Others would be repelled or frightened' (2003: 266). Respondents such as Louis, Justin and John make clear that some individuals can repeatedly fantasise and masturbate about sex with children while having no intention of ever carrying out any such action in real life.

But all in the garden is not entirely rosy. Friday (2003) theorises that men both love women and are filled with rage towards them, and intense rage and sadism certainly do fuel some men's fantasies. Of all the material I have read or watched to research this book – some of which I have had to force myself to look at – there are only three pieces to which I found myself responding with shaking and sobbing, with uncontrollable tears of grief and rage. The first piece at which I cried with distress was the description of young children being sexually abused while timed with stopwatches, given in *Sexual Behavior in the Human Male* (Kinsey *et al.* 1948, discussed in Goode, forthcoming). The second was a series of emails being sent to me over a period of days which appeared to record the behaviour of a respondent, Ian, raping a small boy (discussed in Chapter 10). The third piece concerns the written fantasies of a highly respectable upper-class British man called Roger Took, who was sentenced in 2008 for downloading sadistic pornography involving children and for sexually abusing children in his family. The description of these fantasies is by the journalist Charlotte Metcalf in the British magazine *The Spectator*. This magazine was the only part of the media which recounted in any detail Took's crimes: all other parts of the British establishment remained silent. As Metcalf records:

> The five-year-old girl cowers naked and crying in a corner. She is so frightened that she urinates. One of the men in the room hits her repeatedly. The others laugh. Another man picks her up and throws her face down on the bed. Then the men rape her. She dies soon afterwards of atrocious injuries. This is the scenario that the respected art historian and curator, Roger Took, boasted repeatedly about in internet 'chat rooms' to fellow paedophiles. In the chat rooms, Took relates how a Dutch man bought the child in Cambodia, kept her for a week and how Took was part of the group who enjoyed 'splitting her apart' one night. After Took was arrested last April, the police interviewed him in connection with the child's murder but Took insisted it was mere fantasy and the police passed the case on to Interpol. Fantasy it could be, but the fact so many like-minded men laughed and masturbated over a helpless child's torture, terror and death is chilling and profoundly disturbing. ... on Took's laptop were 742 chat logs of a sexual nature relating to children, adding up to over 1,500 pages. Took posed as 'Dad of 2 Superkids' in the chat rooms and, pretending they were his daughters, posted photographs of his step-granddaughters, Grace, aged nine, and Gillian, aged eleven, comparing their vaginas and inviting others in the chat room to masturbate over the images. ... Again and again, Took and like-minded men salivated and masturbated over the fantasy of raping, punishing, hurting and ultimately killing little girls. ... Took recounted certain incidents, including the gang rape and murder of the Cambodian child and the abuse of disabled three-year-old Cathy [a grand-daughter], with such frequency and consistency that the police treated them as potential facts, but were unable to prove they were not fantasies...One chat log related how

he plied a prostitute with alcohol till she passed out so he could turn his attention to her nine-year-old daughter. Describing with relish how terrified the little girl was as he began to twist her arm before raping her, I noticed the people with whom Took was 'chatting' using the acronym 'LOL' [meaning] 'laugh out loud'.

(Metcalf 2008)

Metcalf's shock and distress at the sadism of Took and his fellow posters is not shared by all. Some professional colleagues of Took's found his 'charm and academic reputation' so plausible that they continued to support him even after sentencing, while in response to Metcalf's article a poster on *The Spectator* site commented:

This article is unworthy of *The Spectator*. What were Took's actual crimes? So far as we can tell, he had pornographic images of children on his computer. It is said he sexually molested Grace. But what does molest mean here? We are told Took got the nine-year-old to pose for photographs. We are not told what kind of photographs. These actions are crimes and Took deserves his punishment but they do not make Took a monster. Mixing in the obvious fantasy of internet chat rooms to suggest he might have been guilty of rape and murder is just ludicrous. It seems the principal victim in this case is Took's wife who is offended that their friends felt more sympathy for Took than for her.

('Don', online, posted 14 July 2008, 6.40 p.m.)

As a society, we find it hard to understand fantasy. Took clearly found pleasure in intensely sadistic and murderous fantasies which most of us would weep even to contemplate: fantasies which, as a wealthy tourist, he was potentially capable of actually carrying out, as indeed he did carry out sexual abuse of children within his own family. It is surprising that a dangerous man like Took is let off so lightly by members of the 'establishment' while, for example, the British actor Chris Langham, similarly convicted in 2008 for accessing child pornography although not for any direct sexual abuse, was excoriated for his behaviour, pilloried in the national press and utterly disgraced in his career. It appears equally paradoxical that individuals such as those respondents in this research project who fantasise only about consensual and even platonic relationships with children (fantasies which, we must not forget, are the standard fare of many mainstream Hollywood movies), are vilified, feared and loathed.

8 Experiences of support

It was such a relief just to discover that I was not alone in loving boys but having no desire to do anything socially/sexually harmful to them.

(Louis)

The fact that my mum has accepted me for who I am even though I am attracted to minors has helped me a lot. I know I would hurt her a lot if I acted out on my fantasies, which by the way I have already promised her I will never do. I would feel I am letting my family down if my self-control fails, they have been real understanding with me and I can't fail.

(Neville)

Having ethical principles is nice, but having friends who confront you with them is better.

(Oscar)

Introduction

As well as getting some insight into how paedophiles develop their sense of identity from the limited range of information and role models available to them, it is also important to understand where paedophiles may seek support – support which may be used either to excuse or endorse offending behaviour or alternatively to assist in maintaining a law-abiding and non-offending lifestyle. We have seen that most of the respondents in this study fantasised and masturbated frequently to thoughts of children, and had typically done so for many years. The question of what support is provided, who provides it and what form such support takes is therefore essential to understanding how some adults sexually attracted to children may choose not to offend.

Two questions were asked on the topic of support. One, in the pilot questionnaire, asked: 'In your own personal experience, which provides most support for you – an online MAA community, or other forms of support? Please describe.' In the main questionnaire, the question was phrased as: 'Where do you generally turn for support if you want to confide in someone about your experiences?'. In addition, people volunteered information in responses to other questions, such as on who they first told, who they would like to tell and haven't, and how their family and friends feel about their sexual attraction. Thus the two main questions on which this section is based are: 'How do your family and friends feel about your sexual attraction to children?' and 'Where do you generally turn for support if you want to confide in someone about your experiences?'

One respondent, Xavier, took the question, 'How do your family and friends feel about your sexual attraction to children?', as literally referring only to the sexual aspect of paedophilia, rather than to the general orientation, and replied, 'To those I have told I did not portray my paedophilia in terms of sexual attraction. That is not foremost in my life. It is certainly one aspect, but not my primary focus. Therefore I cannot say how they feel about my sexual attraction, it is not a topic discussed.' Another respondent, Gus, commented on my question in the preliminary questionnaire, 'it sounds like you are beginning your study with the erroneous assumption that all MAAs are in need of emotional support. This is not the case, many of us overcame that stage long ago and are now emotionally stable.'

Of those who gave answers, some were difficult to interpret in terms of working out whether 'friends' mentioned might be themselves paedophile or not. However, what comes across strongly from the data are the significance of acceptance and support. The role of family and friends is a key part of any individual's self-acceptance. It performs a crucial function in providing a setting which, ideally, can both nurture and challenge us as we test out new ideas and behaviours and integrate them into our self-concept. Where families and friends did know about the respondent's sexual attraction, and continued to support him, this seems to have a positive correlation with a law-abiding lifestyle.

For the respondents in this research-sample, experiences of support varied widely, with five general (albeit sometimes overlapping) patterns emerging:

1. Minimal support: no one knows/support is only from self.
2. Limited support: family and friends know and the reaction has been mixed or negative.
3. Paedophile-based support: support seems to be substantially or exclusively from other paedophiles.
4. Non-paedophile based support: support seems to be available from non-paedophile friends or family.
5. Wider support: support is available from those outside the immediate circle, for example from therapists or the local church. The number of respondents fitting into these five categories is shown in Table 8.1.

It was not always clear from the answers to the questionnaire exactly which of these five patterns some respondents fitted into, as the distinction between 'paedophile' and 'non-paedophile' was sometimes not explicitly drawn. Their quotations have been reproduced for each respondent, to convey the nuances

Table 8.1 Categories of support

Category	Number of respondents
Minimal	5
Limited	12
Paedophile-based	17
Non-paedophile-based	18
Wider	4
Total	**56**

and sometimes the emotional depth of the responses. What emerges in reading through these answers is the sense of a process unfolding over years as individuals recognise their own sexual desires, acknowledge their difference and isolation from those around them, and – over time – reflect on their similarities to, and again perhaps their differences from, others in the online paedophile community. For example, Justin has relied primarily on his own views and beliefs in working out his identity but at times has drawn on the online paedophile community to develop this sense of self, whether in agreement with or reaction against the views endorsed online, while Alan has taken a more active role, choosing to participate and to present his own 'optimistic' comments to encourage 'younger boylovers' online. For those who (willingly or unwillingly) became known to family or friends as having this attraction, ten described negative responses but (perhaps surprisingly) these seemed to be much more about worry or disapproval than outright rejection. The effect of the negative response, however, seems to have been to push the respondent further towards 'like-minded friends'. As Ivan succinctly expresses it, 'many of my new friends are "like-minded", so that speaks volumes. ... this is surely a "natural" reaction of a persecuted minority.' This experience links to those respondents who were clear that their support came mainly or exclusively from other paedophiles. Several respondents seem to have started exploring pro-paedophile sites from a relatively early age; Ed is still only seventeen and Ben talks about telling others online when he was fifteen. As with others, Ben has discussed his attraction with no one else and all his support is from 'ped friends and ped-friendly non-ped friends' he has met online. For families which had already struggled to accept the respondent as gay, the attraction to children was seen as an additional complication which did not need to be mentioned.

Unlike the few respondents who talked about self-reliance in developing their own identities, the twelve respondents who had experienced difficulties with family or friends and the seventeen respondents who looked mainly to the paedophile community for support also appeared to rely on them for a clearer understanding of their own identity and experiences. It was noticeable how often websites, especially online message boards, were mentioned as the main or only source of support, as well as paedophile friends known either online or 'in real life'.

The idea of 'trust' appears again and again in the quotations. In the quotations where respondents talk about why they do not tell their families and friends, the worry about the other's trustworthiness is a reason not to disclose. For those respondents who have told family or friends and have received a positive response, they believe this is because family and friends understand that the respondent can be trusted to keep children safe. In the quotations on limited paedophile-only support, only Ken specifically mentions, under the topics of knowing and support, the fact that 'I've never actually touched any child inappropriately, and don't consider myself to pose any danger to any child'. In the quotations where respondents mention supportive relationships with non-paedophiles, eleven people (Victor, Derek, Gary, Lenny, Vern, Hugo, Neville, Patrice, Pete, Bobby and Louis) all refer – in relation to these topics – to being trusted to keep the law or trusted not to harm children. This is not always straightforward: for example, Hugo's point that his friends 'don't mind as long as I don't hurt or do anything stupid' might mean that support is there to ensure non-abusing behaviour or it might indicate that a blind eye will be turned unless there is egregious wrongdoing. Additionally, of course, it may be far easier to disclose one's attraction to family and friends if one has already determined on a law-abiding lifestyle.

In this chapter, the data are presented according to the five categories given above. Thus, Section I discusses the small number of respondents who reported that no one knows about their sexual attraction, or that their support comes only from themselves. Section II presents data from those respondents who reported that family and friends know and the reaction has been mixed or negative, Section III presents data from those respondents for whom support seems to be substantially or exclusively from other paedophiles, and Section IV from those respondents for whom support seems to be available from non-paedophile friends or family. Section V discusses those respondents for whom support is available from those outside the immediate circle. In Section VI, the chapter concludes with a discussion of the relationship of support to 'contact', that is, to the respondent holding a view that adult sexual contact with a child is acceptable.

Section I: Minimal support

This section presents quotations from those five respondents who reported that no one knows or that they gain support only from their own self. These respondents came across as quite self-sufficient but also at risk of not finding any sources of advice or support when they do feel in need. In addition, although they reported that they did not turn to anyone for support, the quotations make it clear that Justin, Bill and Alan were using the online paedophile community as a source of information and, certainly in Alan's case, were also providing advice to other paedophiles. Bill is the only respondent who mentions considering going to a non-paedophile organisation for support (Stop It Now!, a charity working in child protection), but he is clearly dubious about the extent of help he would find.

I have not told any friends or family about my sexual attraction to children. Right now, I have nobody to confide in about my experiences. I do not trust friends or family. I do not know of any online forums run by non-paedophiles that offer support. And I see little use in confiding with other paedophiles online because I don't think they can see things any more clearly than I can. ... [The online paedophile community] gives me a sense that I am not alone, and that other paedophiles think like me. It has given me new insight into who I am and what other paedophiles are like. Though not dramatic, it has had some importance in my life.

(Justin)

[Family and friends] don't know. I wouldn't turn for support.

(Marc)

Funnily enough I have never got around to telling [my family and friends]. I have come to understand what it is in this life to be your own best friend or your own worst enemy. I have reached a point now where I am confident to rely on my own counsel when it comes to this issue. ... I remember back to the couple of years I roamed around the boy love 'community' on the Internet looking for answers or anything to help me. I didn't find much of any.

(John)

[Family and friends] do not know about it. It is too dangerous to be open about this sexuality right now. [I generally turn for support] nowhere up until now – I am considering joining an online community like [website]. In the real world (offline) there is not really anywhere for MAAs to go or turn to for support (because we are total lepers), except maybe StopItNow, but that is not always suitable.

(Bill)

Never told anyone until I volunteered for an anonymous medical study on the subject matter at NY State Psychiatric Hospital. Never told any family member but assumed that a few may have had thoughts about me. A few friends knew, but mostly I kept it a secret. I have no significant person I wish to discuss this subject with at this time of my life. ... The most important person in my life [as a role model] has always been myself!...I found [website] and enjoy reading and writing in it. [It] is the only web-site I've ever been to that's associated with boylove...[it] has a comforting aspect for me, with the knowledge that there are others who are living a similar life to the one I have had. ... I am very confident in myself and enjoy making optimistic comments [on website] in hopes that they have a favourable impact. ... I feel some good comes out of [site] and it does reassure younger boylovers that they're not alone.

(Alan)

Section II: Limited support

This section presents quotations from those twelve respondents who reported that family and friends do know about their sexual attraction and that there has been a mixed or negative reaction. These respondents, while in some ways less isolated than the previous group, had clearly had some very difficult experiences and seemed to be struggling with finding anyone to discuss their situation with. The lack of support from those around them (while entirely understandable) was clearly pushing these respondents into looking to other paedophiles for a sense of validation and perhaps advice on how to behave.

My mother is mostly worried I will get myself into trouble. Most others either don't talk about it or don't know. [I generally turn for support to] message boards on the Internet.

(Vincent)

They are a bit fearful. [I generally turn for support to a website specifically for paedophiles who are feeling suicidal.]

(Quentin)

Few support me completely, some don't support me at all except for the 'person' I am, and yet many float around in their support of me being paedophiliac. It's hard for them to grasp the concept of paedophilia being a core and fundamental part of my 'self' as any sexuality is. Thus, most will agree with the basic ideology of paedophilia, but are afraid to support it due to stigmatic [sic] or legal influences. ... I usually turn to my paedophilic peers for help and support, if not then friends and family whom I trust in a limited and careful basis; it can get adverse at times.

(Ralph)

My mother doesn't like it, she complains when I look at pictures of child models. She thinks it's sick. Nobody else knows. [I generally turn for support to] online message boards.

(Todd)

The few relatives who know don't talk about it, and I don't have any friends who know. The few I trusted enough to tell are all ex-friends now. [Regarding support] – Are you kidding? I was about forty years old before

I finally communicated with someone for the very first time who had any chance of understanding my 'experiences' and my feelings. Until then, I was in utter isolation. ... Now I have contact by way of the Internet, but the younger ones I can talk to there can't possibly begin to understand forty years of utter isolation, either.

(Eustace)

My mother knows about my attraction range, and 'disagrees' with it. She did not at first believe that my attraction was 'natural', but now she accepts that this is only the case with pre-pubescents. She feels that I could be happy in a same-sex, same-age relationship, but preferably one with a female. She feels that I have been 'groomed' online and face to face by a 'paedophile ring', and that this may be why I express that part of my character. My brother is informed, but has not discussed this with me. I live peacefully with him and my mother. I do not seek support from others.

(Wayne)

My mom hates it. She tries to be accepting, but she always suggests I 'get help' and 'cure' it. I've had better luck with my friends, many of them are attracted to minors themselves, or they're okay with it. [I generally turn for support to] my friends. Always my friends. I can't turn to the Internet, because if I give out too much personal information, I can be outed. If I'm outed, I give up any chance at a steady job or a normal life, and I'm not ready for that.

(Anne)

My mother, the only one of my family to know, believes that it's a harmless phase, but that 'real paedophilia' is a disorder and were mine to continue I should see a therapist. One of my friends is actively supportive (and 'maybe a paedophile' himself), and the others (four) don't care. [I generally turn for support to] the aforementioned supportive friend.

(Freddy, aged sixteen)

[The first person I told was] my father, and he was always supportive. [After arrest for child sexual abuse] members of my family learned about the news, some have rejected me totally and don't want to see me. One of my two families rejected me out of it, while the other one does not know. The friends who know are okay with it in general. However I have recently lost friends, just because they found out I told a seventeen-year-old girl I liked her, without even asking her anything. People are in a state of hysteria right now and it's not healthy. ... [I would like to tell] everyone. I feel living with a secret like this to be heavy and I have enough of living secretly. But with the current climate you can probably understand why. ... I have seen many psychologists...it never changed me or my views on the subject, and I was going there because my mom wanted me to go, I started

at around sixteen or seventeen. [I generally turn for support to] my father, email to some [website] posters (very few and rarely) or [website's] chat.

(Carl)

The answer here is similar to the way Roman Catholic edicts have recently pronounced on gay and lesbians i.e. love the person, hate the sin. [When there were rumours about me] my sister didn't speak to me but eventually, after a few months came round. There has been constant tension with my mom, which I view as a worry she has for me and also a fear of what the wider community in our area will think. But she loves me as a son. I've lost cousins and friends over it, and many of my new friends are 'like-minded', so that speaks volumes. [I generally turn for support to] other like-minded individuals. ... this is surely a 'natural' reaction of a persecuted minority. I have a female friend who has been a great source of support and my family too. But it is mainly to a few like-minded friends that I turn.

(Ivan)

[Family feeling] varies, from supportive to agreeing to disagree. [I generally turn for support to] friends.

(Adrian)

[My family and friends] have totally rejected me and no longer maintain any relationship with me. [I generally turn for support to] other minor-attracted adults whom I know in real life.

(Clive)

Section III: Paedophile-based support

This section presents quotations from those seventeen respondents who appeared to have support substantially or exclusively from other paedophiles. These include one of the three respondents (Ed) who described himself as aged under twenty-one years. Again, as with the previous groups, one gets a sense of fairly isolated individuals finding their only real source of support from within the (mainly online) paedophile community.

The only ones that know about my attraction are my ped friends and ped-friendly non-ped friends (all met online). The only people I have told I have known previously from online ped communities. The first time I became active, telling others anonymously online, I may have been around fifteen, as I recall. I have met several people through these communities that I have met in person and who knew about my attraction. Since I already knew all these people would have been supportive, the response was supportive. But I have never told anyone in real life that I did not know from communities beforehand. ... [I have] no real desire to tell anyone.

There's really no one from my life that I'd like to tell. I wouldn't tell my family since I could not see anything positive coming out from that, and unlike some others, keeping it a secret isn't hard or stressful for me. I wouldn't tell a friend because I wouldn't trust them with that knowledge (nor my family, but I would have more trust for my family). ... I would say [support is provided from] an online community, just because I haven't had experience with other forms of support.

(Ben)

I keep these feelings secret from my family and friends, so I don't think they know. The only support I know of is within online discussion boards where other Adults Who Are Sexually Attracted to Children hang out. If any other support resources exist, I would be reluctant to use them, out of fear that I would be reported for being attracted to children, even though I've never actually touched any child inappropriately, and don't consider myself to pose any danger to any child.

(Ken)

I have told nobody. ['Who are the most significant people you would like to tell and haven't?'] My mother. ... [Regarding the online paedophile community] I enjoy the community and insight of my fellow posters [on website], as well as the ability to talk openly about my feelings. [I visit] several times a day. ... These websites have helped me to understand my attractions to a greater extent, and to understand my place as a MAA in modern society.

(Ed, aged seventeen)

My true friends accept it and accept me. My family does not speak of it. [For support] I talk to my friends who know me and know I am a pedo. Those are the only ones I can trust.

(Max)

Though I think most of my Family (and I mean my GLBT family) knows, it doesn't bother them, because they often leave their children in my care, but it's not out on the table either. If the subject is brought up, it's usually in a teasing manner. My biological family have finally accepted that I am a lesbian after many years, so there is no need to reveal anything else to them. [I generally turn for support to] my diary, and lately [website].

(Bernice)

Friends and family are unaware. [I generally turn for support to] trusted fellow boylovers.

(Nigel)

None of them is aware of my attractions. Internet support boards are currently the only place I feel comfortable talking about it. ... Wikipedia helped me discover that there were people who believed that attraction to children was not evil, and that the predatory paedophiles in popular culture were not necessarily accurate depictions. [Now-defunct website] taught me a lot about who these people are...[the online paedophile community] is the sole outlet for any thoughts I have relating to this part of myself.

(Kristof)

They don't know since I haven't told them. Though undoubtedly there are some among my friends/family that would support me it is still a giant leap of faith. My closest friends suspect, though. [For support] I turn to several people I have 'met' online like on [website] or whatever other board.

(Gavin)

My family does not know. My only real friends are other BL/GLs. No acquaintances know. [I generally turn for support to] other BL/GLs who have become friends over the years. It is with these people that I can express myself fully and freely. Often reading various internet forums such [website] offers support in the fact that I can read experiences that other boy lovers have shared.

(Hans)

Family and friends don't know. It's already difficult enough to assume being gay, I wouldn't want them to know about my attraction to younger boys. I recently met other Boylovers on a board, with whom I exchange a lot. But this is very recent and I usually do not confide in anybody, for there isn't anybody I can talk to about these things. I keep my secrets for me.

(Raymond)

My family and friends don't know about it. I don't trust them with this information. [I generally turn for support to] other 'paedophiles' (adults who are attracted to minors, though some are not paedophiles) who I have come to trust and respect.

(Steve)

I normally turn to online forums for people like me. I also have a close friend in real life that I talk to.

(Xavier)

[Family and friends] are not aware. [I generally turn for support to] the web, e.g., [website].

(Ethan)

I told people online first. Other paedosexuals, and sympathetic people. ... Not counting people I met online, the first person I told was a psychologist. He reacted positively but...he was far more interested in helping me change than in helping me overcome the depression I sought his help for. So I stopped seeing him. [My father] discovered logs of a chat I had with another paedo friend on the Internet, so I had to confess and explain things to him. I wish I could tell my mother, but I know she can't handle it. I wish I could tell my brothers, but I know they would never understand.

(Gus)

[Family and friends] do not know and if they do know about it they do not confront me about it. [For support] I have one person that I talk to and he is very supportive of my desires and attractions. [The online paedophile community] is a very important part of my life.

(Ian)

They don't know, though there is a friend I've been thinking about telling. Obviously, it's a risky situation for us. [I generally turn for support to websites], some place where I can be anonymous, accepted and not always insulted.

(Stewart)

They do not know. [I generally turn for support to] websites.

(Dan)

In addition, one respondent, Samuel, did not complete the questionnaire but gave a recorded interview and described himself in correspondence as largely estranged from his family and heavily involved in the online paedophile community.

Section IV: Non-paedophile-based support

This section presents quotations from those eighteen respondents who specifically mentioned support being available from non-paedophile friends or family. However, as with all the data in this chapter, information is ambiguous and may be put into more than one category. Dirk's quotation, for example, could be categorised under 'Limited support' as it is clear that he did tell his family and the response was negative. It is also not clear that his friends are non-paedophile: thus it is possible that in fact Dirk should be categorised under Section III, 'Paedophile-based support'. However, where respondents have not specified that the friend is a paedophile, it is assumed that they are not.

Family that I have told were quite negative about it and it's a non-issue we never discuss. Friends I have told, on the other hand, are positive and were supportive when I came out. [For support] I mostly go to MAA sites or I talk with friends.

(Dirk)

Only two people know: my wife and a good friend. My wife tolerates me, though clearly she is not happy about the whole situation. My friend is perfectly fine with my sexual attraction to little girls. Our friendship is no different now than it was before I told him.

(Thomas)

My wife, who is fully aware of my BL [boy-lover] nature, is the most important support I have. Online groups count for nothing compared to her. ... [The most significant people I would like to tell but haven't are] my daughter and her husband.

(Frank)

Nobody in my family or friends knows about it, except my best friend. He sees nothing wrong with it as long as I do not act illegally or immorally, which he trusts me not to, rightly. [I generally turn for support to] online communities, mainly [main boy-lover site].

(Victor)

*My mother I told shortly before she died – she was very accepting and understanding about it. ... She told me she had known for years that I loved Little Girls...She even showed me some photographs of herself as a Little Girl that I had not seen before, and told me a fascinating story about her own father – how he had once told her (when she was a young woman) that he had not only loved her as a child, but had been **in love** with her; she told me she thought it was all very beautiful and quite romantic. Other than that, I have told only two friends (I mean real life, offline friends). One I told more or less by accident. ... He is a trusted friend, whom I've known for years, and while he was certainly not positive about paedophilia, he was able to divorce that from his view of me, and it did not affect our friendship. The other friend reacted similarly...I once asked him why he thought, as he viewed paedophilia so negatively, that it had not affected his opinion of me or our friendship at all adversely. His reply was: 'Because I know **you.**' [I generally turn for support to] [website] and also to people I have got to know on that site, whom I can talk with by way of email. Occasionally, also to the friend I mentioned above, though not often as I usually get the feeling that he would prefer not to talk about it.*

(William)

My family probably has strong hints about it, for I don't really hide my attraction at all. My friends have actually been quite supportive. A few have gotten bad reactions, namely from when I dated a nine-year-old. They are mostly very supportive, and seem to accept that it's just a part of who I am. [I generally turn for support to] my friends, actually. I do a bit of stuff online, but I find most of it to be rather impersonal.

(Ulf, aged sixteen)

They're not happy about it, but they're generally loving and supportive. [I generally turn for support to] message boards or the Internet.

(Andy)

At age seventeen I found the online BL community. I told these people about my feelings. My mother knows, and most of my friends (five people). The first people I met in person, who had similar feelings as mine, served as role models for about two years. [My family and friends] all trust me to do the right thing, but feel extremely uncomfortable talking about it (one exception, though). It leaves me with the feeling they still accept me as the person I've always been, but not as the paedophile I've come out as. [I generally turn for support to] fellow paedophiles, the Internet. I mostly try to support myself, though. I don't like being dependent on other people.

(Derek)

I told a good friend of mine first. He was largely accepting, as he'd known me quite a long time and understood that I was not a child molester. He did have a lot of questions and later he was a bit disturbed by it and we got into a serious debate by way of e-mail. He still accepts me and has been the one steadfast friend through all the shit I've dealt with since then. I broke down and told him sometime around my last year of college, when I was extremely depressed, was on the verge of suicide and needed someone to talk to. It was before I became aware of [a girl-lover board]. Everyone in my family and all my friends know, and pretty much everyone in my community has become aware of it. Obviously, being that I'm out and had a webpage for a while, it wasn't too difficult to find out. [My family] had trouble with it at first, particularly my sister. Now that they realise I'm not a child molester they are much more tolerant and accepting. Some of them may not understand it, but they have never outright condemned me or cast me out of their lives because of it. [I generally turn for support to] either through the arts or on one of the [girl-love] forums I belong to...My goal is to seek acceptance for those with my orientation.

(Gary)

I can't say they approve, but they have been supportive. My arrest made it impossible to keep that particular cat in the bag. My parents were there for my trial (1,500 miles away from their home). I have a warm relationship with my parents as well as my sister and brother and their kids. There have been rocky moments from time to time, but overall they have been very understanding, if not approving. [Despite having online support] I do feel a real lack in this area. I'd very much like to have a more personal relationship with another boylover. Someone with whom I could share my everyday thoughts and feelings on boy-related subjects.

(Jerry)

My [family] all accept my feelings, but my feelings (and how I cope with them) are never openly discussed. Their acceptance does not mean they approve or even understand, but they know that I would never harm a child. I have several friends who also accept my sexual orientation, and two in particular (life-long, close friends) discuss with me in some detail, my predicament, and the unjust way that society treats paedosexuals. [I generally turn for support to] my two life-long friends, as stated above.

(Lenny)

I'm out to one person, they don't seem bothered by it. [I generally turn for support to] that person, or online forums.

(Oliver)

My family, as such, does not know. My girlfriend knows, but she feels that as long as I'm not breaking the law, it should be okay; earlier she tried to get me to go to a psychologic [sic] treatment, nevertheless the doctor stated that there's nothing much she could do about it, and I should not really be worried about it either, as long as I don't actually try to do something illegal by the letter of the law. I don't have many friends (say, four or five), of them only one knows; he is sometimes making fun of me for it, but that's it – he finds it more humorous than problematic.

(Vern)

Two friends know and don't mind as long as I don't hurt or do anything stupid. [I generally turn for support to] myself. Generally never turn to others for support.

(Hugo)

Friends do not know about it, and my parents do and have taken it pretty well saying that as long as I treat the kids well and do not break the law I should not worry too much about it. [For support] I can talk to my mom as she is real open-minded and she is now used to listen to me talking about my sexual attraction to little boys, she is real good with me and provides me with support. ... The fact that my mom has accepted me for who I am even though I am attracted to minors has helped me a lot. I know I would hurt her a lot if I acted out on my fantasies, which by the way I have already promised her I will never do. I would feel I am letting my family down if my self-control fails, they have been real understanding with me and I can't fail.

(Neville)

My family doesn't know about it. My friends neither, except for one female friend of mine to whom I told everything a few weeks ago and who accepted the idea very easily. The key is to know the person very well: she knew and still knows that the last thing I would want to do is to hurt a child, therefore she trusts me entirely. Of course, I have several boylover friends but I don't think that counts;) [For support] there are not a lot of possibilities. I go quite often to forums to participate in discussions. That's where I met a few boylover friends who are now real-life friends and on whom I can rely. The best solution is to talk about it, whether it's on msn or in real life; try also to seek advice with the older members who had their share of joy and disappointment and who probably experienced what you are going through right now.

(Patrice)

[The first person I told was] a psychotherapist I began seeing after a suicide attempt, he was sympathetic and helped me accept my feelings and stop judging myself. ... [I have told] one or two family, several friends. ... Otherwise, no one really. As I get more confident with expressing my feelings, people are beginning to understand for themselves. Support and acceptance from my friends is infinitely more valuable and meaningful to me than online support. I find online relationships somewhat vicarious and abstract.

(Tim)

Section V: Wider support

This section provides quotations from those four respondents who discussed having support available from those outside the immediate circle, for example from therapists or the local church. Clearly, these respondents are in a minority in the sample, and it was very interesting to read about their unusual experiences.

I can write a book about it. I tried to be as open as possible. I came out first to my best friend. She was very understanding and tolerant. After that I told my parents. They reacted just the way I thought ('We somehow knew it, but never mentioned it – we hoped you would grow out of it...') But they accept it now. We talked about it. My father read a book about it (which I recommended) and my mother took me to some meetings. They are sometimes very concerned about me. With other friends I see two different reactions: first is they accept it and start to reinterpret the subject of paedophilia. Second is that they start to act like a shrink. They want to 'help' me. Happily that doesn't happen often. ... I am not alone. My wife is standing beside me, even if necessary my parents. Also my Christian faith helped me through difficult times (especially during teenage years). Having ethical principles is nice, but having friends who confront you with them is better.

(Oscar)

My daughter accepts it, but sees it as a problem; she trusts me concerning my behaviour. [Family]: they accept it, and me as I am, seeing it as a problem *that I never may and can do what I might want to do. They trust me concerning my behaviour. Friends within the ped-community: they accept me completely and sometimes see me as a counsellor or a model. We can speak freely. Friends outside the ped-community: They accept me as I am. We can speak more or less freely. Neighbourhood: accepts in various grades from 'not' to 'okay'. Contacts for example in my church – some know. They **tolerate** me under certain conditions, but do not really **accept me as I am**. [I generally turn for support to] the ped-community in which I have good friends.*

(Pete)

My friends do not know about it, except the paedophile friends I've made online, a few of them I've met 'in real life'. I revealed my attraction to my family (parents and brothers) a few years ago, when I went through a deep depression. I am lucky they took it better than I expected (or rather, feared). Especially both my parents. They've displayed great support at once, even if they had a long way to go from helping me in my depression to understand my attraction, one turning-point being when, under my insistence, they started to separate my illness (clinical depression) from my sexual identity. I think it opened their eyes on many issues too. They constantly remind me how much they trust me, they know I would be incapable to harm a child. If they are concerned about me, it is not because of me but because of the dangers, worries and solitary life I have to face. [For support] I began a therapy about the same time I outed myself to my family. I disclose everything to my therapist. I also talk to my parents, but I avoid the most worrying topics to protect them. But the people I talk the most to are a few other boylovers like me, on chat, and sometimes IRL [in real life], even if most of the time I'm more their confidant than they're mine. But I like that role.

(Bobby)

The example of Louis exemplifies the experience of a man who has felt able to ask for support and help and who has received it from a number of people, both those in his immediate circle and more widely.

I am quite out in my community and always have been. I am not an activist or advocate of intergenerational sexual relationships. All my close friends and family know about my sexuality. All of them without exception have trusted me around their children. I have a policy of never being alone with other people's children, but this is more for my protection and their peace of mind than out of any real fear of temptation. My friends/family are disturbed by the nature of my sexuality, they don't like to hear much details, but they have always trusted me to be dealing with it and as one of my friends said to me, 'I know you and you are not a predator'. I have found my friends and family to be supportive of my struggle, a surprising

number have actually 'come out' to me as having similar feelings them-
selves at times (though mostly towards young girls). ... I have a number of
support networks in place. First I have God and my church family. ...
Second I have my friends. Like the Church mentors they support and
accept me, but really don't have a clue how to help me. Third I have been
to many counsellors. ... They have also helped me to accept myself and
manage certain attitudes and behaviours in a healthier manner than I was.
Finally I have my online MAA community. ... Before I met these guys I
was quite suicidal. They have helped me and been such a hugely influential
force for good in my life. Through them I've come to better understand and
accept myself and my sexuality. It was such a relief just to discover that I
was not alone in loving boys but having no desire to do anything socially/
sexually harmful to them.

(Louis)

Section VI: The relationship between support and 'contact'

I initially hypothesised that the more non-paedophile support an individual
had access to, the more likely they would be to hold a 'non-contact' position
in relation to sexual contact with children, and conversely that the more
paedophile-only support an individual had, the more likely they would be to
be open to the idea of sexual contact with children. I also hypothesised that
this relationship might be subject to age, so that the older an individual was
(and thus the longer he had been exposed to a paedophile milieu) the more
likely he would be to endorse a 'contact' position. These hypotheses are not
borne out by the findings from this small study.

In order to devise a form of words which did not ask people to incriminate
themselves in any way, I decided to use the term 'non-contact'. This term was
chosen after discussions with Claire Morris (a doctoral student researching in
this area) and Dr Richard Green (her doctoral supervisor and a well-known
academic in this area). Unfortunately, the question 'Would you describe
yourself as "non-contact"?' led to a number of respondents either mis-
interpreting the question to mean 'Do you avoid any form of contact with a
child, including social?', or simply stating that they did not understand the
question. Although clarification was obtained from some respondents in a
follow-up questionnaire, this could not be done with all respondents and
made interpretation of the findings difficult. Those who gave unclear answers
are not included in the following analysis.

Leaving aside the three youngest respondents and those whose attitude to
sexual contact with children is not known, there are three subgroups of
respondents: those aged twenty-one to thirty (twenty respondents); aged
thirty-one to forty (fifteen respondents); and aged over forty (nine respondents). Of the forty-four answers to the question on contact, there were
twenty-one who gave a clear 'yes' to the question 'would you describe yourself

as non-contact?'; twelve gave a clear 'no'; two stated that they were currently non-contact but had not always been; and nine stated they were non-contact in practice but in principle agreed with sexual contact with children, for example writing, 'I do not, or have never, engaged in sexual contact with a child. However, I consider myself pro-contact, because I think the laws should be changed to allow some sexual contact between adults and children' (Todd). No clear pattern emerged in relation to age. No doubt if I had been able to interview these respondents face to face, or explore their written views in more detail, it would have been possible to tease out some more of the nuances in their attitudes towards sexual contact. As it was, I was constrained by the requirement not to ask incriminating questions and it is likely some of the respondents felt similarly constrained in their replies. Hence these findings should be regarded as highly tentative until further research is done. However, it is intriguing, for example, that of the thirteen respondents who referred, in the previous section on fantasies, to the distinction between 'fantasy' and 'reality' and the need to control or manage their fantasies, all but one (Max) stated that they were non-contact (n = 9) or non-contact in practice (n = 3).

If the five forms of support are divided into two broad categories: those with non-paedophile support (including the 'non-paedophile friends' category and the 'wider support from the community' category) and those without non-paedophile support (including 'self', 'mixed' and 'paedophile' categories) the figures for those supporting a non-contact position are almost equally divided between those with and those without non-paedophile support (ten respondents with non-paedophile support versus eleven respondents without), and similarly the figures for those holding a 'yes, but' position on non-contact are also almost equally divided (six respondents with non-paedophile support versus five respondents without). The only clear difference is in the number of respondents answering 'no' to the question 'Would you describe yourself as non-contact?' Of the twelve respondents answering 'no', only one (Vern) had non-paedophile support. The other eleven answering 'no' had either paedophile-only support (n = 7) or 'mixed' support (n = 4).

What these very small-scale and preliminary findings seem to suggest is that those who have no support outside the paedophile community are more likely to agree with sexual contact with children, while those who have sup-port available from non-paedophiles are more likely to hold 'non-contact' views. Clearly, it is easier to talk about your sexual attraction (and garner support) if you can insist that you do not intend to break the law and harm children. However, the relationship may also go in the reverse direction – that, if you are able to talk about your feelings in a supportive environment, you may be more likely to continue to accept the mainstream view that sex with children is wrong, and also be more able to turn for support under stress so that you are able to maintain non-offending behaviour. Nevertheless, it is also noticeable that seven of the twenty-one respondents who hold non-contact views were seeking support *only* from other paedophiles, whether online or IRL. This therefore lends support to the suggestion that some paedophile communities may be working successfully to encourage non-offending. As one respondent, Bill, commented, although he relies primarily on himself and does not seek outside support, 'If the question means am I non-contact in a sexual sense, then yes I am. I follow the ethics that can be found on most online paedophile communities.'

Considering the question of acceptance and support, as presented in these quotations, it is clear that most people have a very circumscribed experience of support, which is often drawn solely from the paedophile community, typically online. Even where other sources were available (for example, from accepting family or friends) it still seems from the responses that the primary source of support remains other paedophiles. With a small number of respondents citing 'no one' as their source of support, and an equally small number being able to ask for support from a range of sources including non-paedophiles outside their immediate circle, the great majority of individuals in this sample could look only to other paedophiles to understand and share their experiences and feelings. Thus it would seem that, in this sample, sources of support outside the paedophile community are considerably less common than those from within the paedophile community. This is of course an unsurprising finding given the level of secrecy surrounding the experience of sexual attraction to children, but the implications for those struggling to construct and maintain a law-abiding lifestyle would seem to be potentially major.

The next chapter follows on by looking at some key issues currently being debated within the paedophile community. It is important to remember that, if an individual has nowhere else to turn to discuss his feelings except to the online paedophile community, these are the debates and the views he will be confronted with and, as this chapter has demonstrated, many adults sexually attracted to children are likely at present to receive most or all of their advice, information and support from the paedophile community.

9 Debate and dissent within the online paedophile community

Some place where I can be anonymous, accepted and not always insulted.

(Stewart)

The largest danger facing members of my community is isolation and lack of accountability to those around them. The current environment allows the radical viewpoint on each side to hold sway, rather than involving community members in efforts to find solutions that meet the demands of accountability to others.

(Darren)

Controversies over 'contact' are one of the most common threads on [the main discussion board].

(Tim)

Introduction

There is perhaps no better way to introduce this chapter than to reproduce two comments, by Darren and John, on the felt rejection by 'straight society' which may lead some paedophiles to question and then in turn to reject social norms and laws.

I would certainly not celebrate my condition, though (if one can approach the subject impartially) it does have redeeming merits. We are motivated, by nature, to involve ourselves in the lives of children, and often-times those lives are difficult and abusive. We are characterised as being 'exploitative' for such endeavours. I have twice in my life spent my own funds to travel for extended periods of time to areas of the world subject to utter poverty, and to build and work in orphanages; few of those who find me evil incarnate find time to help the purported objects of their attentive gaze. We find straight society to be very hypocritical.

(Darren)

A person with this attraction is in a real sense pushed out of the community. He can end up feeling he's unwanted and not a part of it in any way. If he's outside the community and its laws then what laws does he abide by? What laws cover him? An example, so there's a ten year old boy outside my front door kicking a ball around. Society has an almost biblical hatred for me because I have this attraction. If I open the door and make contact with the boy and something sexual arises from it, then society will have an almost biblical hatred for me then too. So what's the difference? Damned if I do, damned if I don't. Can you tell me why I shouldn't open that door? Society and its laws fade into the background for a lot of people with this attraction specifically because the community has no 'grace' for anyone with this attraction. There is nothing I could ever do to be an accepted part of the community. They have no laws that express my right to exist, my right to friends, family or dignity. So do I create my own laws? Do I then follow them as strongly as society does even if they're in conflict?...I remember back to the couple of years I roamed around the boy love 'community' on the Internet looking for answers or anything to help me. I didn't find much of any. I remember seeing some things written on bulletin boards that I thought were sick. Sometimes it angered me somewhat as I was beginning to blame people who wrote things like that for making society hate me even though I did nothing wrong. But I couldn't write anything in response to them because I also had this same attraction and at the time my 'moral compass' was shattered along with everything else inside me. ... I couldn't say anything because it also felt like the 'pot calling the kettle black': 'Who I am to criticise anyone?' I turned my face away, haunted by the shame of inaction and paralysed by fear.

(John)

This chapter explores the ways in which the online paedophile community responds to differing opinions on key topics. In this chapter, Section I outlines some of the relevant aspects of the online paedophile community, including questions on 'contact' and the impact of anonymity. Section II explores the range of respondents' attitudes to child pornography and visual imagery of children, and Section III examines what respondents said about the relationship between using fantasy, using visual imagery, and acting on one's fantasies in real life.

Section I: Aspects of the online paedophile community

We have our own language, our own customs, our own websites. That's a community.

(Gus)

As is clear from the previous chapter, the online paedophile community often plays an important role. As William commented, if Internet sites were to be closed down:

> *I am certain that the community is now so well-established at its core that it would survive – somehow. Even if the very worst happened, and we could have no forum of any kind, the spirit of the **core community** would remain, even if we could only email each other. And we would do everything we feasibly could to re-establish ourselves. … some would suffer from a lack of support. And it can never be good for people to feel isolated and alone. There will always be occasional individuals who find it hard to steer a positive course through life without good sources of guidance and support structures from among people like themselves, perhaps because they don't have any other means of communing, or due to other personal factors/disadvantages. So we do need these communities, and it is important that they remain.*

Online pro-paedophile discussion boards often have discussion 'threads' which debate issues concerning legality, ethics, and political responses to sexual attraction to children. A key finding from this study which needs to be emphasised is that there is no monolithic, homogenous 'view' held by all paedophiles. Instead, there is a spectrum of views ranging, for example, from acceptance of the kinds of evil so chillingly depicted by Roger Took (see Chapter 7), to an absolute adherence to celibacy and a fully law-abiding lifestyle. A moderator of a major site wrote to me:

> *This forum provides the means for a community to develop, for [paedophiles] to interact with each other, question each other, discuss ideas, form bonds, provide mutual support. … we operate scrupulously within the law. Law enforcement agencies are fully aware of the existence of our sites and doubtless monitor their content closely. Strictly speaking, every poster on [this site] is 'non-contact' – because no poster is having illegal sexual contact with underage girls. (As far as this is possible to know – stating such would be against the rules of the forum. But I do **not** believe any of our posters are behaving illegally in their private lives).*

Stewart made the point, 'Even in the MAA community, we disagree on key issues, such as AoC [age of consent] and contact' and as Tim noted in an email to me, 'controversies over "contact" are one of the most common threads' of discussion on the major pro-paedophile discussion boards. These controversies are both philosophical and practical. As Bill pointed out when discussing his 'non-contact' position, 'I follow the ethics that can be found on most online paedophile communities' but of course most discussion boards do indeed follow an overt 'non-contact' policy, if for no other reason than the pragmatic one that if they are seen to advocate criminal behaviour the website would be closed down. The 'pro-contact' and 'anti-contact' positions are debated regularly, and the key points of these two positions were explained to me as follows:

> *'Pro contact' means to take the view that, while a person wisely obeys the law, in principle, laws aside, there is nothing wrong with loving and*

consensual sexual contact, and therefore to argue for changes to the law. This seems to be the opinion of the larger section of posters. It is important to stress than none of these advocate breaking the law: they simply argue for a change in societal and therefore legal opinion. There are many shades of opinion within this: some feel the AOC should be lowered, to varying degrees; some have other ideas about different legal arrangements...and some feel that there is in principle no need for any legal restriction on children behaving sexually. It is important to note that this is all seen from the point of view of the moral rights of children and young people.

There are others who are 'anti-contact', to differing degrees. These are a smaller section of the community, but they feel that it could never be right for children and adults to act sexually with each other. Of course they may express that to different degrees and with different shades of emphasis. Very occasionally...someone pops up on the board who argues that paedophilia in itself is negative: that is, that [paedophiles] should seek therapy, and so on, to rid themselves of the attraction itself. This is a very, very rare viewpoint among [site users], and other members of the community – I think quite rightly – will argue strongly and passionately against it. The pro and anti contact arguments are a different thing; there is a mutual respect there (if sometimes a little grudging!), an acceptance of the person alongside a vigorous and lively debate about the arguments.

(Moderator of major pro-paedophile website,
personal communication)

Ben exemplified the debates and tensions caused by this when asked if there was anything that particularly concerned him about pro-paedophile websites:

People on there that are obviously pro-contact, have no reason not to have sexual contact with children, and obviously do not care about the welfare of children...[It's] the BS [bullshit] factor...it's obvious to me that some posters have sex with children, but of course would never admit it and would deny it or skirt the question if asked. I hate superficiality and lying so that's one part of [the online paedophile community] I don't like.

It is therefore difficult to know, simply from reading the public postings on the boards, what the attitudes of individuals posters may be and whether any claimed adherence to a law-abiding lifestyle is merely a cynical 'front' to enable continued web-presence or whether it is a genuine and deeply-held ethical position.

Another factor mentioned by several respondents was the impact of anonymity on posters' felt need to take a responsible stance. When individuals post anonymously, they cannot be held to account for anti-social or irresponsible postings. Individual posters may be 'flamed' or criticised, and as a last resort may be banned from moderated sites, but those who argue persuasively and persistently, for example for the 'right' of young children to 'sexual experience', will find a hearing online which they might never receive through any other medium. This irresponsible behaviour by a small minority may have the effect of distorting the public debates to make the 'online paedophile community' appear far more radical than it actually is, as the 'silent majority' lurk and read but do not contribute. This can be true for many online communities but is perhaps particularly so for paedophiles. As discussed in the previous chapter on 'support', the online paedophile community plays a tremendously important role in the lives of many paedophiles today and many may feel loath to disrupt that sense of support by criticising others online. Respondents explained to me that there is little wish to cause difficulty in the one place where you feel welcomed, where you go to feel 'accepted and not always insulted' (Stewart). There is a sense that, with everyone feeling so beleaguered already by 'society', it feels wrong and even disloyal to criticise anyone's views. As Oscar explained:

> *I used to write often on a moderated site, an online community. But most of the time people wrote about how nice their trip to the swimming pool was, how handsome their boyfriend is, how lonely they feel if their buddy is gone for holiday and so on – if you ask a critical question, people start to curse and condemn you.*

Oscar chose to rely instead on 'real-life' communities where 'the communication is more open and real. The content is often very deep. We discuss for example how to deal with family, what about coming-out, how do you accept your feelings, what about faith and religion and so on.'

Tim also expressed ambivalence about the value of the online community and hinted that boasting might not be unknown:

> *It's useful for me to post there, because I felt so lonely with my feelings for so long, but I don't agree with everything said there by a long shot. ... You also have to remember that a lot of these people have suffered a rather intense attack by society on what is for them a core aspect of their being. Rejecting society's attitudes and opinions is for many a survival strategy. ... A lot of paedophiles talk big about kids and sex, but I doubt many men who were having sex with children would go bragging about it in a public forum. The Internet isn't that anonymous.*

Perhaps also, as John suggests, paedophiles may believe they have no *right* to challenge or criticise others, as it may feel 'like the "pot calling the kettle black": "Who I am to criticise anyone?"'

The online paedophile community is of course not alone in struggling to develop and maintain a positive sense of itself as a coherent entity. Many factors militate against the creation of an online 'community' among any group of people, whether that is through bulletin boards, message or discussion forums or social networking sites such as Facebook, MySpace and so forth. Computer-mediated communication (CMC) is frequently described as encouraging spontaneity, non-conformity and even disinhibition – a mixed blessing as this can lead to increases in both friendly, intimate disclosure but also hostile verbal attack (Reid 1999), and as we have seen from the respondents' remarks, hostile attack online, where people may 'curse and condemn you', can be acutely wounding for those already feeling vulnerable. In order to be more than simply a conglomeration of individuals visiting and posting on a site, a 'community' needs to have stability over time, and investment in constructing and maintaining the shared social space. Social cohesion and some level of control need to be present, usually provided online by web-editors and moderators. Just as in the physical world, the online 'community' is largely imagined, an emotional investment in a shared vision (Anderson 2006), and as the quotations from the respondents make clear, their online social networks do not exist in isolation but alongside other significant networks and relationships, with a small number of respondents having relationships which crossed between 'online' and 'IRL'.

Online communities, with their inbuilt safety net of anonymity and the security of knowing that most participants share one's specialised interests, can provide enormous emotional support as well as advice, companionship, reciprocity, allegiance and a sense of belonging (Wellman and Gulia 1999). They can be, at their best, a warm and caring space. For paedophiles specifically, as we have seen, the online community may provide the only support they have for reflecting on their sexuality. Wellman and Gulia (1999: 187–8) see a significant characteristic of online communities as their 'glocalised' nature: they are simultaneously global and intensely local, where the individual is 'usually based at their home, the most local environment imaginable, when they connect with their virtual communities…community has moved indoors to private homes from its former semi-public, accessible milieus such as cafés, parks and pubs.' This aspect of 'community' again engenders a sense of privacy and even secrecy, despite the very public nature of Internet postings and the paradoxical intimacy formed with strangers online.

While the anonymity of online postings offers the benefit of egalitarian comradeship as well as the problems of disinhibited spite, lack of accountability or irresponsible claims-making, anonymity itself is a formidable barrier to any genuine sense of 'community' emerging. We can only form associations or relationships with people whose reputations or merits we can assess in some way, usually by knowing them over time. Donath (1999) differentiates usefully between pure anonymity, in which we can know nothing about an individual, and pseudonymity, in which a stable reputation can be built up over time. This is clearly the case in the online paedophile community, in which pseudonymous identities may last for decades and, as 'old hands', can be regarded as offering support and wisdom to 'newbies'. As noted earlier, in Chapter 6, at least four respondents from this research were cited by other respondents as having been influential to them, and there is evidence of the usual cliques, leaders, followers and hierarchies of influence in this community as in any other.

Within the online paedophile community, in common with other online special-interest communities, we find a spectrum of affiliation and engagement and a mix of support, self-absorbed obsession, boasting and 'flaming' (responding angrily to others' postings). What may particularly distinguish the online paedophile community is its emphasis on anonymity and pseudonymous identities. This provides freedom to abdicate accountability in expressing political or other views, while at the same time the community is constrained by an emotional pressure to be non-controversial and to avoid criticising others who are likely to be feeling as isolated and vulnerable as oneself. The result of these two conflicting forces is likely to produce a false sense of consensus, as people feel able anonymously or pseudonymously to put forward extreme views which others then feel unable to publicly challenge or disagree with. This posited false sense of consensus is important because of the online paedophile community's status as a major source of information and support. While there may be many 'lurkers' who post nothing but only read others' contributions, there appear to be a fairly limited number of constant members with a high presence and thus a high level of influence in setting the tone of debates, and this again may contribute to the development of narrow, inward-looking views and a limited sense of possible areas of discussion and debate. Thus the views propounded on the Internet and the views actually held by many paedophiles may be significantly discrepant.

In order to go at least a little way beyond the tensions and superficiality of some of the online debates, I asked the respondents to comment on a number of controversial topics including attitudes to child pornography, child sex tourism, sexual contact between adults and children, faith and religion, age of consent, and the ability of children to consent. I also asked about their role in community and political activism, what they felt the 'online paedophile community' should do in mediating and endorsing particular views, and the relationship between the 'paedophile community' and 'society'. For reasons of space, this chapter can explore only one of these issues in any depth. The chapter will therefore focus only on one key debate, which is the attitude to child pornography and the related question of whether using visual imagery increases or reduces the likelihood of acting on one's sexual attractions.

Section II: Attitudes to child pornography

In [some] forums, people are encouraged to view barely legal photo gallery sites. I think that's a bad thing and it could easily serve as a gateway to truly illegal pornography and it's an invitation to porn addiction. That is, of course, not a good condition to find yourself with when the porn you are addicted to could land you in prison or warp your mind to the point where you might consider acting in an inappropriate way with a child. ... [my advice is] don't get into porn because many people do and don't get out until they are in prison.

(Gus)

It starts off looking at what society generally deems as relatively normal pictures that are contained within 'boy love community' sites. Those pictures are rarely updated. Over time the person can end up branching out and basically combing the Internet looking for more pictures and more 'revealing' pictures. It will only be a matter of time before they are standing at the front door of a child pornography site. This was as far as I got...thankfully I was working my way out of that blind misery by the time I reached that serious point and basically just switched off the computer and never went back.

(John)

On the main questionnaire, one of the questions posed was, 'In society, generally, there is a lot of concern over child pornography. What do you personally feel is appropriate regarding visual imagery of children?' Again, the question needed to be worded carefully to avoid asking anything incriminating, such as 'Do you yourself use child pornography?' The same provisos therefore need to be applied here as to the data on sexual contact with children. Answers varied in length, with three respondents (Steve, William and Tim) providing two to four pages each of detailed argument. The responses by the three under-age respondents are excluded. Other than the under-age respondents, forty-six people gave answers. The responses can be broken down into a number of categories. I have summarised these in the following nine statements, with the number of respondents shown in brackets:

1. It's a plot to prevent people knowing the truth about child sexuality (two).
2. It's a plot to stop paedophiles enjoying themselves (one).
3. It should be okay to view pretty much anything, with the possible exception of coercion (three).
4. Showing kids having fun sexually and consensually is fine (fifteen).
5. It's not wrong so long as money is not involved (four).
6. Producing child pornography may be wrong; viewing it is not (eight).
7. Nudity without explicit sexual content should be legal, as should material in which no child was involved (e.g., cartoons) (nine).
8. The current legal situation is about right (two).
9. It's a difficult dilemma and understandable why someone would find themselves using it (two).

The responses therefore clustered around a broad acceptance of some, milder, forms of sexualised visual imagery of children, with thirty-six of the forty-six respondents sharing this view; six respondents apparently holding a more libertarian view and only four respondents holding a more 'mainstream' view.

Within the broad consensus, there were different emphases on the question of consent. A number of the respondents felt that it should not be illegal to possess (and possibly to share) a drawing of a child or a photo of a nude child taken with their consent and not for profit. Most respondents felt that the question of consent was important, but this came across as being more to salve their own consciences than genuinely to protect children. They appeared to believe that a child would be able to understand what it would mean over the long term to have sexually explicit pictures of themselves globally distributed or sold on the Internet, and that they would be in a situation where they could freely consent to (or refuse) such an invitation. They also appeared to have a naïve idea that pictures taken 'not for profit' are qualitatively different from commercial pictures and that there would be no overlap between those two categories. Some respondents also appeared to feel that they could distinguish between children genuinely 'having fun' and those who had been told to smile at the camera. No respondent mentioned any age, intellectual capacity or other limiting or coercive factor which might make it more difficult for a child to give or withhold consent, or any minimum age below which they believed a child would not be capable of giving fully informed consent.

1. It's a plot to prevent people knowing the truth about child sexuality

I wonder if the banning of child pornography is not to keep the people ignorant and to continue to spread lies. … Sure there is exploitation but I believe the other side of the medal exists…and might be much greater and more beautiful than the one we almost if not always see.

(Carl)

I believe, if a couple of ten-year-olds want to perform 'sex play' in front of a web-cam and share it with the world, this should be legal. … Some children enjoy the exhibitionism of it. … I will come right out and say, that I have outwardly advocated the return of child pornography to its former status of being legal. I continue to advocate this, today. … The real motive behind keeping visual records of childhood (and intergenerational) sexuality hidden from the public is to…help complete the socially imposed illusion that children are not sexual beings [and] to provide an easy manner in which to apprehend and imprison non-violent members of a sexual minority. … I would agree, however, that it is in bad taste and very disrespectful to keep pictures and movies of a person actually being raped, brutalised and/ or murdered. … Had today's technology existed when I was a kid, I can almost guarantee you there would be 'child porn' movies floating around the Internet today with me in them, at the age of ten, eleven, twelve, maybe even younger. It is something which appealed to me when I was a kid.

(Steve)

Although only two respondents gave answers which referred to this idea of people being 'prevented' from knowing about child sexuality, this view seems quite widespread among some members of the paedophile community. To some extent, it underlies work by the Kinsey Institute and those who have subsequently made use of the Kinsey data, for example Floyd Martinson

(1973). We also find it expressed more recently online by the Dutch activist Norbert de Jonge, who has written:

> I'm using Child Love TV as yet another tool in trying to convince the world that...everyone should *accept* their pedophilic feelings...You realise how absurd it is to even have to explain the benefits of greater sexual freedom for children, when you see a child – when you see child pornography of consensual sexual contacts. ... This, of course, is one of the reasons why anti-pedophiles want *all* child pornography to be illegal.
>
> (de Jonge 2007, emphases in original)

This view has clearly had some level of impact, and leads to a situation where at least one respondent, Steve, does not stop to question why or how two ten-year-olds would decide to 'perform "sex play"' and 'share it with the world'. Steve also does not notice that, in fact, when he was growing up, there may not have been 'today's technology' but there were certainly both still and movie cameras, so the assertion that it 'is something which appealed to me when I was a kid' and it was only lack of technology which prevented him from participating seems more like an adult sexual fantasy than an actual recollection of reality. Altogether, the views on children's sexuality portrayed in these quotations say far more about adult sexual fantasy and wishful thinking than about a genuinely child-centred view of the world.

2. It's a plot to stop paedophiles enjoying themselves

> *I think the 'concern' isn't so much about protecting children from harm as it is about preventing paedophiles from having anything they could get any enjoyment from. ... Age is completely irrelevant in any moral question, only the desires of those directly involved are relevant. ... If [the image] appears to be professionally produced, for profit or otherwise, and everyone in the image is clearly aware the image was being made for distribution or publication, and there is nothing in the image suggesting force or coercion, then there is no reason to restrict publication or copying other than ordinary copyright laws.*
>
> (Eustace)

Here, Eustace provides a view which comes across as typical for him. He tends to have a resentful and almost paranoid approach to life, no doubt in part arising from his experiences as someone who does seem to care about children but who feels unable to express his caring in a socially approved manner. The notion that anti-pornography laws are simply a way to make life difficult for paedophiles is one which also comes across in Steve's comment that the real motive is to 'provide an easy manner in which to apprehend and imprison non-violent members of a sexual minority' rather than to protect children from abuse.

3. It should be okay to view pretty much anything, with the possible exception of coercion

Everything should be able to be viewed.

(Derek)

Anything legal for any other status.

(Adrian)

Any imagery is appropriate other than obvious forced sexual imagery.

(Hans)

These very brief quotations indicate that, for these respondents, the question of child pornography was not one about which they held particularly strong or carefully thought-through views. For people who structure their lives around the idea that children are central to them, and who claim that, as a group, they are more in touch with children's well-being than the average person, I found myself surprised when respondents appeared to be simply not interested in questions of children's welfare or child protection.

4. Showing kids having fun sexually and consensually is fine

I abide by the law in these matters, and would advocate doing so. ... If the viewer or downloader is contributing in any way at all to 'supply and demand' then he had better be certain that the picture was taken under the best moral conditions. Because his actions are having a consequence. ... If they have deliberately chosen to look at, or 'get off on', a picture which they know contains harm, then this is one seriously sick and twisted individual. ... An erotic picture depicting happy children, and taken with their consent, I can see no harm in. ... I myself certainly had sexual feelings from a very young age. I know that I was masturbating from the age of seven or eight.

(William)

I believe that society should transition and accommodate child erotica; a benevolent form of child sexuality and sexual expression. ... It is inhumane to disallow an eleven-year-old boy from having his own form of erotica to masturbate to. ... Why should we fear a paedophile having access to child erotica if it within itself is non-problematic?

(Ralph)

Many people who view or collect child pornography pose no harm to society. I also feel that children should not be abused or harmed in the making of such visual imagery, but I also feel that sexual activity in itself does not necessarily constitute harm or abuse.

(Ken)

I don't really see the problem as long as both the boys and the adults are consenting. Of course, the boys have to be willing to do what they're asked to do.

(Patrice)

As long as the child is not hurt or distressed by the making of such visuals. ... and from there on, actually protecting her from society doing harm, if the original act is found out.

(Vern)

As long as no one is being hurt and they have said yes it should be okay. Adult magazines have not increased sex crimes against adults, so why would child porn?

(Max)

I believe if whoever is on film is having a good time there should be no issue with its production or viewing.

(Quentin)

A depiction of a child, nude or scantily clad, is acceptable, even if sexually posed. ... they [the children] should be allowed to consent to the pictures being taken [and then not released until the child reaches age of majority]. I don't believe any child should be forced to do something they don't want to and parents should be part of the decision. ...

(Stewart)

I only advocate viewing of material which is produced with the full consent of the child, which the child is adequately compensated for and which the child is aware will be made available for distribution.

(Clive)

Child pornography should be forbidden only when it is (probably) the result of an illegal sexual act.

(Vincent)

I believe that the 'naturist' photos found in my possession were beautiful images; and that material produced with the consent of the subject is harmless. Pornography in my opinion is material where consent was not given or where pressure or power has been exerted, or where actual harm to the child has occurred.

(Nigel)

As long as all parties participating agree I see nothing wrong.

(Hugo)

[Nude images should be legal.] Since children are allowed to masturbate, pictures or videos of children masturbating should be legal. ... The child and/ or the child's parent or guardian should be giving consent for the production of such images. ... 'Internet child modelling'...should be fully legal.

(Thomas)

Should not be criminalised. The only thing that should be illegal is causing direct harm to someone. Viewing, possession, distribution and so on – none cause direct harm. **Production might** *but only if coercion was involved, in which case it falls under the criteria of causing direct harm to someone.*

(Ethan)

Photographers such as Jock Sturges, David Hamilton and Sally Mann have stunningly captured the beauty of children. I also have little problem with photographs that are more sexually explicit though I would take into account whether or not the children posing/modelling are doing so with consent. ... Better stay with the likes of Sturges or Mann.

(Gavin)

As can be seen, this view was the most typical. It reflects in part the confusion in wider society over what constitutes child pornography and what is merely erotic art portraying children, or the acceptable commercial use of images such as photographic modelling by models under the legal age of sexual consent. There is a suggestion, for example in Gavin's answer, that paedophiles may use mainstream photographic work such as that of Jock Sturges to masturbate to: this may provide an acceptable legal outlet for sexual-tension release.

5. It's not wrong so long as money is not involved

It is only inappropriate if the child suffers. Once disseminated, I have no objection to even the worst material, if it is not paid for. Most children do not suffer in the making of CP [child pornography]. Many of them make their own, and it is often only the fools who label it pornographic.

(Wayne)

The personal ownership of **any** *image of* **any** *type should not, in itself, be a criminal offence, providing that the images were not bought, requested or traded.*

(Lenny)

All situations where children feel at ease can be photographed, but private or personal situations are best left in private photo-albums. Personal pictures are of no concern to other people.

(Dirk)

*I don't think just viewing child pornography should be illegal, because really, you're arresting people for thoughts. If someone **buys** child pornography, or requests someone make an image, yes, they should be punished, but not as severely as the child pornographers themselves.*

(Anne)

These quotations illustrate what appears to be a highly naïve view of the world of child pornography. Remarks such as the acceptability of 'even the worst material, if it is not paid for' suggests, absurdly, that the most vile abuse of children would be acceptable if it takes place in a non-commercial environment, presumably committed by the child's family or carers (and see Jim Bell's comment on this, below). The further comment that most children 'do not suffer in the making of CP. Many of them make their own' also reflects a view of the world entirely at odds with the reality portrayed, for example, in the quotations given in regard to Freenet (Leurs 2005) and other Internet sites (Jenkins 2001).

6. *Producing child pornography may be wrong; viewing it is not*

I do not think it should be illegal to possess.

(Todd)

To possess CP is a thought crime (Orwellian)…but if you produced the material (especially the serious stuff, that is, rape) then the law is right. Nude photos and lower end stuff especially if the young person is participating I don't see a problem.

(Marc)

I don't believe people who look at these images should be prosecuted. People who produce those images should be prosecuted, if the images are truly abusive.

(Andy)

I feel that producers of child porn should be arrested and 'put away' for a long time. I believe those caught with child porn should be arrested, but I feel the penalty for possession is far too high, as it is predominantly a thought crime (unlike production, where children are directly involved). … [Children should give consent when over the age of majority, and images of them should then either be legally registered or destroyed].

(Gary)

I do not feel mere consumption is harmful, but production involving children definitely is.

(Victor)

I don't like the idea of possession of images being illegal, and in no other crime are they. Law enforcement resources would be put to better use seeking out those who committed the crimes depicted rather than imprisoning anyone who happens to view them. That said, I understand the aversion to the images, especially if what law enforcement says about many of them involving violence is true. But I don't believe that simple child nudity should be lumped together with such images. These should be legal, and not in the grey area sort of way that some of them are now.

(Kristof)

As I have no desire to now engage in a sex act with a child, the viewing of such material is no more likely to cause me to do so than listening to an Ozzy Osborne album is likely to cause me to commit suicide. … I have a difficult time believing that many of the children who appear in such media are willing participants, that is, free of coercion of some sort. … for the protection of children I feel pornographers should be actively hunted and imprisoned [but] if it's already out there it shouldn't be a crime to possess it. [Artwork] should be fully legal.

(Jerry)

Personally, I would regard a work like 'Show Me' by photographer Will McBride as a cultural treasure. … I have no problem with depicting child nudity or sexual activity, but I can't dispute that sexually abusive images of children do exist. For many of these, perhaps the only harm is in a betrayal of privacy and trust, but this in itself cannot be trivialised. Fetishising sexual situations involving children in internet pornography is only tangentially related to paedophilia. … The capacity for sexual arousal to children is very common, and novelty is a powerful erotic stimulus. All kinds of men fall down this particular rabbit hole, as news reports continually remind us. … I don't think it's blameless to collect abusive images of children, but I think I can understand how easy it might be to get entangled in something like that. … If children are abused in the creation of an image, then the manufacture is illegal and should be punished if possible. If acquisition of an image contributes to its creation, e.g., through financial exchange, then some culpability falls on the acquirer. … [but] 'making' here [in the legal context of downloading] is a synonym for looking, and to avert one's gaze is not necessarily a moral act. … the law has succeeded in creating a common marketplace, blurring the boundaries between appealing and repugnant, and providing links from one to the other like a trail of crumbs…If taking simple pleasure in the sight of a nude child is a terrible crime, what a small step it then becomes to taking pleasure in the sight of a child masturbating or having intercourse, and where is the line between that and a child being raped? Children are sexual. Where's the harm in acknowledging that? If we can't, we have no way of identifying abuse, and that's what puts children at risk.

(Tim)

Many of the comments given here resonate with concerns shared by members of society generally. The 'particular rabbit hole' of viewing child pornography, as Tim reminds us, is one which appears to be a widespread problem and is not by any means restricted to self-defined paedophiles. Perhaps the most highly publicised international police operation to date on child pornography offenders has been Operation Ore. In Britain, over 7,000 men were arrested, and one of these, Jim Bell, wrote about his experiences:

> For three years, as an internet consultant, I collected child pornography off the web and saved it to disk. I used my knowledge of the Internet to find it, from the mildest to the most extreme. ... The worst child pornography is free, posted on news servers by individuals who want to share their interests with others. By this I mean pictures of small children forced to engage in sexual activity with adults. ... My own experience suggests that many of these men [using commercial sites] did not believe, or did not allow themselves to believe, that they were guilty of using child pornography. As commercial site users, they were not downloading the extremes of child pornography...
>
> [On commercial sites] There was a very clear distinction between American and European artistic sensibilities. American sites would feature the girl next door, in a bikini or a sexy little outfit, looking like a fashion model or a pop star. European sites would favour nude little girls indoors or outdoors, singly or in groups, with a high standard of photography. ... But the intention is to provide men with masturbation fantasies of young girls: in the case of Candyman [the main site investigated by Operation Ore], reportedly 250,000 men worldwide. ... Hardcore is not the name of this game. It means that it was fatally easy for 7,000 men to convince themselves that looking at pictures of heartbreakingly pretty little girls was not wrong. It is why I do not find it surprising that men who enjoyed teaching children, or keeping them safe in society, should have enjoyed such pictures. We obey laws most easily when they fit our own instincts of right and wrong. When they do not, we tend to finesse and rationalise our actions. We have an infinite capacity for that. In prison I met perhaps 100 men who had been convicted of offences against children. None of them admitted that they were paedophiles – none. The social stigma is too appalling. I cannot admit what I am to myself. ... None of us use that word or even admit to ourselves the thought. ... The sexualisation of children through television, pop music and fashion is acceptable, it is done for fun: the world of internet child pornography merely completes that process.
>
> (Bell 2003: 2–3)

In this quotation, Bell makes the surprising assertion (which I have not seen elsewhere) that the worst pornography is free and it is only the mildest which is available commercially, although this situation may have changed since

2003 with the increase in live webcam sex for sale. Bell also describes vividly how the men downloading sexualised images of children did not regard this as child pornography and did not identify themselves as paedophiles. It is clear, from the quotations presented here, that it is still very difficult to reach an agreed social (if not legal) consensus on what is and what is not child pornography.

7. Nudity without explicit sexual content should be legal, as should material in which no child was involved (e.g., cartoons)

> *The laws are far too harsh, but I'm unsure as to the related morality. Simple nudity should probably be considered acceptable.*
>
> (Oliver)

> *It depends on the purpose of the person creating the image. A parent taking a picture of his or her child running around naked because it's cute is okay. Someone taking pictures of real children for the purpose of sexual arousal is wrong, in my view. I also think that possession of such pictures should be a crime. I do know, however, that sometimes telling the difference between innocent and erotic images of children can be difficult. To me, taking pictures of blatant sexual activity involving children is harmful, but when it comes to pornographic cartoons and 'virtual porn', I am not so sure. There are good reasons for it to be both legal or illegal.*
>
> (Justin)

> *Simple solo pictures of children in nude shots is fine but anything that shows an adult having sexual relations with a child is not good.*
>
> (Ian)

> *For a paedophile in the current times, what's appropriate for him is to abide by the law, whatever it is. What the law **should** be, though, is different than what it is in some places. As for sexual contacts, informed consent is essential. But the problem with a photo or a video is that you can't know the story around it. So graphic documents with kids should remain illegal to prevent abuse as much as possible. But nudity in artistic shoots, or on a naturist resort are a whole different matter. In some places, graphic drawings aren't legal either, while no kid could have been harmed in the process, which demonstrates that it's not the production of image that is aimed at, but the fantasies themselves. This is the most dangerous misconception one has to face on the issue.*
>
> (Bobby)

> *I do not have any wish to look at child pornography because I really would not get any pleasure out of seeing the ones that I love the most being hurt, degraded and abused. Even if it looks like the children are enjoying taking part in it, I do not feel that child pornography is ethically correct. ... I do not*

have a problem with ordinary nudity (e.g., naturism). ... I also do not see anything wrong with ordinary images of clothed children.

(Bill)

Non-sexually explicit images of children in the nude or partially clothed is acceptable to me. However I do not believe depicting sex acts with minors is appropriate. A child posing provocatively does not seem harmful (for the child) to me. I do worry about any child being coerced into this situation, though.

(Xavier)

I don't like the idea of sex with children being viewed by anyone. However, I think nudity is beautiful, and if the child agrees to be filmed in an atmosphere where nudity is accepted and enjoyed then that should be perfectly fine... roaming in the woods, playing volleyball on the beach, things like that.

(Bernice)

I do not need any (child) pornography and I am against it. It violates the privacy of a child. Only on strong conditions (consent) nudity can be pictured. Cute clothed children may be seen.

(Pete)

Any photos taken in which children are being engaged sexually are inappropriate. Even if the photos in question do not show the actual sexual activity. If children are not being engaged sexually, then I am open to a wide variety of child photography, including nudes. However, if any image of a child causes the viewer to be aroused then I would say that looking at that image would be questionable for that individual.

(Louis)

A number of the quotations presented here are closer to the mainstream understanding of child pornography. They also begin to engage more closely with the question, not just of the represented child to the image, but of the recording adult to the image and subsequently the viewing adult to the image. For Justin, for example, the nature of the image changes dependent on the sexual intention of the adult recording the image, and for Louis, it changes dependent on the sexual arousal of the adult viewing it.

8. The current legal situation is about right

The current legislation on this point seems good to me. I am opposed to the merchandisation of the child's body. I identify it as a kind of rape. Even though those who should be punished are the 'producers' more than the 'consumers'.

(Raymond)

I do not like pornography as it makes the little boys look filthy which they are not. ... It is fine [remaining] illegal as it is.

(Neville)

Only two of the forty-six respondents appeared to consider that current legislation has achieved the correct balance in this complex situation. This is a surprisingly small number. This may be because other respondents, who implicitly agreed with the law in general, did not agree with the stance on nudity. Common sense might suggest that we would not expect paedophiles to feel that child pornography is wrong but, as we have seen from the comments in this section so far, the situation is far from clear-cut and many respondents in this sample hold views on child pornography which, although they are not in line with national legislation, are still not as far from mainstream views as one might originally have predicted. I will close this section with two comments which highlight the complexity of this subject.

9. It's a difficult dilemma and understandable why someone would find themselves using it

Well, I see it as a dilemma. Child pornography is wrong, ethically unacceptable and I know many paedophiles are addicted to it. I used it myself too, felt not free and destroyed it. It makes your mind troubled. What you see is what you want. On the other hand it can be a medium to use for discharge your sexual desires. Personally I doubt about that; non-pornographic pictures can do the same. Although I prefer nudist pictures (I'm sure others would call them child-pornographic as well).

(Oscar)

Life can hurt beyond words, every day, every week, every month, every year without reprieve. ... What's left of their psychology can end up huddling around the last 'feel good' factor left within them, which of course is the [sexual] attraction [to children]. Attraction basically works by releasing feel good hormones...reducing stress, reducing blood pressure and basically has a soothing effect. ... Looking at pictures can end up being used as the psychological equivalent of taking a Prozac. ... Over time they will need more and stronger doses of it. It starts off looking at what society generally deems as relatively normal pictures that are contained within 'boy love community' sites. Those pictures are rarely updated. Over time the person can end up branching out and basically combing the Internet looking for more pictures and more 'revealing' pictures. It will only be a matter of time before they are standing at the front door of a child pornography site. This was as far as I got...thankfully I was working my way out of that blind misery by the time I reached that serious point and basically just switched off the computer and never went back.

(John)

In this research, five respondents mentioned the term 'addiction'. Lenny, in Chapter 5, mentioned that he had been addicted to child pornography (for which he had been sentenced). In Chapter 10, Ian talks, not about pornography, but about his sexual addiction to small children. Oscar and John (and Gus in the quotation heading this section) talk about the dangers of becoming addicted to child pornography. The compulsive escalation of the search for more, and more extreme, images is something which is widely discussed in connection to child pornography (for examples of the literature in this area, see Taylor and Quayle 2003; Quayle and Taylor 2005; O'Donnell and Milner 2007). While it is clear that escalation of use, leading to a form of psychological addiction, is a problem for many individuals, the evidence from this small sample of respondents provides some tentative indication that such escalation does not always occur and that some individuals at least are able to recognise the dangers and self-regulate their use of images. The next section goes on to explore how respondents thought about the relationship between their use of visual imagery and their behaviour with children in 'real life'.

Section III: The impact on real life of using 'visual imagery'

Given that most respondents considered that it was probably acceptable to possess at least nude photographs or graphic drawings if not actual ('consensual') sexually explicit images, what impact did they feel this had on their behaviour in 'real life'? Clearly, I could not ask any respondent directly if they themselves used child pornography, as this would be an admission of criminal behaviour. I therefore asked about the use of 'visual imagery'. Among the seventeen respondents who were asked two follow-up questions on the issue of the relationship between fantasy, using images and acting sexually towards children in real life, there was, not surprisingly, a range of views on these questions as well.

Of these seventeen respondents, unexpectedly, only one (Justin) was quite clear that 'having sexual fantasies about minors would make someone more likely to act on their attraction to minors, in my opinion' and he felt that this was also true for visual imagery, while one (Patrice) was equally clear that fantasy and relationships are not related, stating baldly:

> *It is not linked at all. Having sex with a minor is not about fulfilling a fantasy (or you're a real pervert who's going to hurt the child), it's about having a relationship, a mutual one. A boylover doesn't 'act' on a fantasy, he acts if a lot of conditions are fulfilled. [Images are] only linked probably for rapists or murderers, who are people who act on instinct. Let's not put everyone in the same basket!*

At the other extreme, Raymond, who does not describe himself as non-contact, gave the equivalent of a shrug to the questions:

I suppose you're talking about paedophiles fighting their paedophilia, wanting to have no fantasies. I have no problems with my paedophilia. I am happy with it. And the other paedophiles I know are like me. So I don't know. ... I personally don't use imagery of minors, but I know most paedophiles do. ... But I don't think it's wrong to have sex with children.

The other fourteen respondents who were asked these questions all gave variations on the view that using masturbation fantasies or images could lessen the likelihood of acting-out one's fantasies in real life. For example, Pete commented, 'For me, and others to whom I have spoken, fantasising helps to keep hands off. ... For me, I only very seldom see pictures, but others, who see them frequently, say it helps them to keep hands off.' Bobby answered, 'My experience proves that it didn't make me more likely to act on them. ... As for other people, I bet many people are like me. ... The link between a fantasy and an act is much more loose than people are prone to assume.' Kristof commented, 'I would say less. It can serve as a release for feelings that would otherwise build up and become an obsession.' Marc, having used child pornography, was clear that it had 'done the total opposite and relieved the stress and frustration', while Stewart was less sure:

it does both in my opinion and experience. In my case it helps me to be less likely to act though that makes it sound as though before them I was going to no matter what, which is untrue. ... it can have the reverse effect where you fantasise so much you start to believe it and are more likely to act on it.

Louis gave a thoughtful and careful response, distinguishing between fantasising about known and unknown boys:

I haven't fully decided what I think about this. I think it is important not to sexually fantasise about boys I know in the real world. I'm sure that if I used boys I knew in my sexual fantasies that I'd be inclined to think more sexually about them when I was with them. ... I guess I don't believe that fantasy will make me act out in the real world. I also find that regular masturbation (which inevitably includes boy fantasy) helps me control my sexual cravings and thoughts in my day-to-day dealings. I think if I spent my time fantasising that I could actually have a real sexual relationship with an actual boy then it may well encourage me to go after making that fantasy a reality. In my opinion, this goes beyond fantasy into actually hoping and planning (which I think often pre-empts actions of some sort).

Similarly, Oscar emphasised the importance of not using images of boys known to him:

I'm sure that if a person has sexual fantasies and feeds them thinking about a boy he knows, the step towards acting on them is smaller. In my opinion (and experience) it is safer to minimise sexual fantasies about someone you know. ... if I use visual imagery of minors, my fantasy is being focused on boys I don't know. So that's rather safe. If it were photos of boys I know, it could be more of a problem not to act sexually. On the other hand, if those visual images contain pornography, the sexual component of my feelings is being stimulated. I think you should not stimulate the sexual component, nor ignore it. There must be a balance between both. This balance could be using non-pornographic nude-boy pictures. But I know from others that they have a different balance-system.

Neville had a much more pragmatic response. He felt that the only reason to choose imagery over action in the real world was to do with the probable consequences, and that if 'the consequences or punishment for looking at imagery and acting out on them are the same it is better to act out on them...in an ideal world we would stay away from both, but ideal worlds do not exist.' On this aspect, one respondent (Ivan) discussed with me the fact that possession of child pornography is often a straightforward crime to prove and therefore convict for, while actual sexual abuse of a child is very difficult to prove. Thus, in his experience, paedophiles might be likely to weigh up the chances of being caught for using pornography versus being caught for sexually touching children – and might decide, unlike Neville, that the relative risks made direct sexual contact the safer bet.

On the whole, however, the view which came across in this sample was that the internal constraints of personal ethics would be the most likely factor in determining if fantasy led to action. Jerry, for example, expressed it as:

I believe that fantasies about minors can lead to trouble for people who are troubled, but that it wouldn't make any difference at all to a true minor-attracted adult who was aware and accepting of their sexuality and aware as well of the consequences of such an act. ... I don't see any difference between mental or visual imagery. Is visual imagery supposed to have an impact of increased magnitude? Certainly not to my thinking.

This chapter has indicated the wide range of opinions which are held by this one small sample of paedophiles on the controversial subject of child pornography. In this way it is hoped that this study can help to undermine the view of the 'online paedophile community' as a homogenous group sharing identical views, and can begin to highlight, and contribute to, dissenting voices within the paedophile community which argue for a genuinely ethical and law-abiding stance to children and sexuality.

10 What stops adults preventing the abuse of children?

> The significant problems we face in life cannot be solved at the level of thinking that created them.
>
> (Albert Einstein, attributed)

Introduction

Research has much to say on why children find it difficult to report abuse: for two of the major texts in this field, see Driver and Droisen (1989) and Cox *et al.* (2000). It is not hard for us to understand the many reasons why a child cannot name what is happening to them, does not understand that this is not 'normal', does not realise that other adults should be there to protect them, and cannot find the courage or the opportunity to speak out. But that leaves many questions unanswered. What was happening to the adults around that child, who may well have suspected what was going on but who did not intervene? What was happening to the adult abuser, who knew that what was happening was wrong but who did not seek help to stop?

This chapter explores those two key questions. The first section is a case study of Fred, a man who learned that a friend of his was accessing online child pornography. This case study illustrates some of the consequences which happen when an adult does decide, against many social norms, to take action and report a colleague to the police. The second section uses the case study of Ian, a paedophile with whom I corresponded as he appeared to agonise over whether or not to report himself to the police for his sexual offending. The case of Ian gives an insight into the mind of a man who knows, on some level, that what he is doing to children is destructive and abusive and yet who is too frightened of the likely consequences to seek help in stopping the abuse.

(All names in this chapter are fictitious, some identifying details have been changed and some of the material has been edited for brevity and clarity. Other than that, the material given here is presented exactly as it was written to me.)

Section I: Why don't adults report abuse? The case study of Fred

This case resulted in a man, Tommy, being convicted of possession of many hundreds of images, some showing children as young as six or seven years old. As well as links to 'hard-core pre-teen' sites, Tommy had apparently also accessed pornographic web-cams and was also suspected of having sexually abused girls who were the children of women he had partnered. Tommy was discovered because, while he was staying in a colleague's house, child pornography was discovered on his computer disks. The colleague, Fred, reported Tommy to the police and later corresponded with me, discussing the case as it took place over a period of months. The extracts below are from Fred's correspondence with me, as he struggled to deal with the consequences of having contacted the police, and the impact this had on the university department where they both worked.

> *At first I had no concerns or suspicions about him. Although I had seen him form an extremely close relationship with the daughter of his previous partner I never suspected anything untoward in this. ... I remembered going to visit Tommy one day. ... I remember ringing the doorbell and being surprised that it took so long for anyone to answer. [His partner's young teenage daughter] answered in her dressing gown. She told me she was off school sick. Then Tommy appeared and we chatted and I left. I thought nothing of it until I began to be concerned about Tommy's increasing closeness to [another teenage girl]. ... [when the child pornography was found] I was dumbfounded. I didn't know how to respond. After all, he was my friend, my colleague at work, and living in my house. I also worried that, if I told the police, they would say I was involved as it was happening in my house, since he was downloading this stuff through my internet connection, accessing these sites with an ISP number that could be traced to my name. I discussed it with my wife, who suggested I confront Tommy. I chose my moment and told him what we had found on his computer disks.*
>
> *The implications of what has happened seem to keep expanding as more people are dragged into its orbit. At the university there seems to be two reactions.*
>
> 1. *Denial. People who were informed but chose to do or say nothing. It also appears that there have been scandals in the department in the past that were covered up. Some of these people were involved and to them I am a troublemaker.*
> 2. *Looking out for themselves. Some people as I told you were directly involved and now need to justify and explain their (in)action. To them I am also a troublemaker.*
>
> *I made a statement [to the police] and handed over the disk I had found. Tommy's house was raided and he was arrested on a charge of possession of objectionable material. This happened some months ago. The police told me that he admitted visiting child porn sites and 'inadvertently'*

downloading some porn from them. They encouraged him to plead guilty and enter a program they have running for such offenders. However he has refused this much as he refused my offers of help. Instead he has begun a line of action that is almost unbelievable. When you consider that I know what he is and he knows that I know his behaviour is chilling. He has begun a relationship with [a woman]. Since his arrest they have got married and she is now pregnant. His family has rallied around him. He has name suppression. After his first court appearance he returned to work and told no one. He obviously intended to continue as he had before and just brazen it out. I informed the Head of Department about what was happening and he was supportive to an extent. He told me I had done the right thing but no one was going to thank me for it. This has proved true. Tommy has been suspended from all duties until the matter is resolved. This however has been put about by Tommy as the motivation for me trying to set him up because of professional jealousy. Throughout the time while waiting for the case to go to court, Tommy has been playing the part of the victim and maintaining his story that my daughter and I had maliciously set him up. His explanation for his guilty plea is that as a young, newly married man, whose wife has just given birth, he cannot afford the expense involved to clear his name.

There is more I could tell you but as you can imagine I am tired of it. I feel I have become as isolated as he has and am on trial as much as he is. It is possible he will get off. I will be disappointed but can accept this as I have done something and not protected and enabled him. Whatever happens I will have marked him and he will not have the freedom and cover he has operated under. But I have been marked too and realise the university wants to be rid of me as much as him. My position at the university has become unbearable.

As you might understand I have little sympathy with paedophiles. I can't understand the extent that people protect them. Not only people within his family, who must know, as he has to my knowledge conducted at least two relationships with young girls in front of them. But also people who have been victimised by him – [the woman] whose daughter I believe he had sex with when she was twelve seems to have forgiven him and is supportive. My wife seems to hold no grudge against him even though he brought this stuff into our house and left it around for [our children] to see.

Tommy arranged a meeting with the Head of Department where he informed him that he had retained the services of a top lawyer, that the case would be thrown out and after that he would pursue a private prosecution against me for laying a false complaint. This story was given credence and passed around the Department where it seems it was largely believed. The distance that others were establishing was not in my imagination but very real.

If you report a paedophile then you are held in equivalence with them. At the university we have both been given the same sort of treatment. He has been told he cannot work there until this has been settled. I have been told that there is no work for me. If he is found not guilty he will be welcomed back – it will justify all those who did nothing. If he is found guilty I won't be asked back. The elephant in the room all the time that was never mentioned, although it was presented with the evidence, was what had been found on his computer.

You must remember that my original concern was about his behaviour with children, not his use of pornography. I had already begun to suspect Tommy of grooming and seducing children, and finding the pornography was just another confirmation of these suspicions. I felt that I had found him out but that I had no solid proof. I thought that the disk was enough to confirm suspicions but it was the paedophilia, not the child pornography, that I was concerned about. However, I thought the disk was not enough, I had no material proof that it was his and it would be my word against his. Other people I told about it agreed and were content to know about it and take no action. But I could not let it rest. I felt that as I knew what he was doing, I was responsible to try to stop it. Telling people at the university who were in positions of authority, senior members of staff, was an attempt to, if not pass on, then share this responsibility. It was only when they took no action that I finally approached the police. I did this to share my concerns and try to shed this responsibility. I was concerned about his behaviour with children; the disk was the only evidence I had beside my own word.

When the police said they were going to prosecute him over the disk I was horrified. I thought that it would come down to his word against mine. I wanted to pass on my knowledge of his behaviour and have someone with more authority than myself look into it. Still, I felt that I had done the right thing. Even if he was brought to trial and got off – something that would rebound very unfavourably on me – I had at least acted and tried to stop this abuse of children. I was prepared to live with this, as I had found the alternative of keeping quiet to be unbearable. It was not until the police showed me a record of what had been found on his computer that I felt some relief. He had continued to access child pornography sites and download videos of children being abused up until he had been arrested.

[Eventually Tommy was convicted and sentenced.] So he never came back to the university. No one has said anything to me on an official level. Despite the facts above being known he still has his supporters. I have been told *[a senior staff member]* openly supports him when the topic comes up among staff members. This senior staff member knew about the disk I had found before I contacted the police but remained his strongest supporter. The comment on what has been found on his computer was that it 'shows how bad my timing was. It was a few months ago that he found his partner was pregnant and since he has since married her and hasn't downloaded anything since, it shows he has put this all behind him'. This from a senior academic and one who witnessed firsthand his obsessive relationship with *[a girl]*, who would have been twelve at the time. Also, when his computer was confiscated by the police, it was found that he had been accessing hardcore pre-teen sites up until the day he was arrested so it is obvious that there

was no way he had put this behind him once he started his new relationship.
I feel that he was not charged with the real offences he had committed
and think that he is still a threat. It was a weird experience being forced
out of the university. However, I do not regret what I have done. I believe
now that there are situations when, like it or not, you have to do something.
The people who want to get rid of me are those who chose to do nothing
and I remind them of this.

Fred found out at first hand some of the pressures which keep us silent about our concerns and which then, when we courageously do decide to contact the police, contribute to our feeling ostracised by those around us. A backlash by those around us occurs against our speaking out because it exposes those facts which we would rather not confront, the atrocities in our midst. Our speaking out challenges both those who abuse power and those who stand by as muted witnesses, and the responses of those around us send a powerful message that it is better to remain silent and not disturb the status quo. This is true in many other 'whistle-blowing' contexts, in which as a society we often have an ambiguous attitude, arguing for the necessary legal protection to 'speak truth to power' while at the same time frequently resenting or even despising the unfortunate person who does break confidentiality as being a 'sneak' or a 'grass'. In cases involving unpleasant subject matter such as sexual abuse, our feelings are often even more ambivalent and there is a sense of not wishing to attach one's name, and certainly not the name of one's institution, in any way to something as unpleasant as 'paedophilia'. This means that there is a strong urge to keep matters 'in-house' and avoid police intervention. There is also a reluctance to believe ill of anyone and perhaps also to admit that one might have been wrong: that the person previously valued as someone decent and friendly could be capable of such harm. Additionally, in the early twenty-first century, with the recent history of 'moral panics' over 'false memory', 'Satanic abuse' and other perceived hysterical overreactions to the threat of sexual abuse, there may be a particular reluctance to be seen to overreact and thus actually to respond in any way. The routine psychological and bureaucratic mechanisms for smoothing over scandals come into play.

It is easier, as Fred found out, to side with abusers than to serve as effective witnesses to the abused. Even in a case as clear-cut as Tommy's, in which it was incontrovertible that images of severe abuse had been found in his possession, there were nevertheless those who preferred to continue to think of Tommy as a 'good bloke' and Fred as the jealous and resentful troublemaker, just as the wife of Roger Took (discussed in Chapter 7), when she spoke out about his abuse of children, found herself sneered at by Took's colleagues as being 'jealous' of her 'younger rivals'.

The psychiatrist Judith Herman, Professor of Clinical Psychology at Harvard University Medical School and a pioneer into the study of Post-Traumatic Stress Syndrome, has studied the issue of social responses to perpetrators of abuse, whether those perpetrators are state-sanctioned torturers, violent husbands or sexual abusers of children. She has found that, in any context of abuse:

> It is very tempting to take the side of the perpetrator. All the perpetrator asks is that the bystander do nothing. He appeals to the universal desire to see, hear, and speak no evil. The victim, on the contrary, asks the bystander to share the burden of pain. The victim demands action, engagement and remembering. ... In order to escape accountability for his crimes, the perpetrator does everything in his power to promote forgetting. Secrecy and silence are the perpetrator's first line of defence. If secrecy fails, the perpetrator attacks the credibility of his victim. If he cannot silence her absolutely, he tries to make sure that no one listens. To this end he marshals an impressive array of arguments, from the most blatant denial to the most sophisticated and elegant rationalisation. After every atrocity one can expect to hear the same predictable apologies; it never happened, the victim lies, the victim exaggerates; the victim brought it upon herself, and in any case it is time to forget the past and move on. The more powerful the perpetrator, the greater is his prerogative to name and define reality, and the more completely his arguments prevail.
>
> (Herman 1992: 7–8)

Fred, as the bystander who chose to take action, finds himself made the scapegoat in the place of the actual perpetrator who is protected, and in the absence of the actual victims who are largely invisible and silent. How often does this almost-ritualised dramaturgical response to disclosure play out in communities? We cannot know, as it is seldom captured in conscious realisation or articulated as carefully as Fred has been able to convey. Nevertheless, it appears to be a significant response to disclosures of abuse and this may well play a key role (along with loyalty, embarrassment, shame, doubt, and indifference) in why adults aware of abuse may choose not to report their concerns, or may be ridiculed and silenced once they have.

Section II: Why don't abusers seek help? The case study of Ian

Having looked at some reasons why those around the abuser may not report abuse, the second part of the equation is the abuser himself (or herself). Ian exemplified this situation of a sex offender who appeared to seriously consider seeking help but then drew back. Ian is the pseudonym of one of the self-defined paedophiles who contacted me as part of the MAA Daily Lives Research Project. He got in touch in 2007, completed the main questionnaire and offered to stay in touch. I then asked him to complete some follow-up questions which he did at the end of 2007. I thanked him for his contributions and expected that the correspondence with him was now closed. Instead, in 2008 he got back in touch and began to write to me in detail about his sexual attraction to babies and young children. The correspondence continued for a few months and then came to a close. During the correspondence, as I became increasingly concerned about the behaviour he discussed, I reminded him several times of my role as a researcher and drew his attention to the research Information Sheet (Appendix B) which stated that, if a respondent disclosed previously unreported criminal behaviour and I could identify that respondent, I would report them to the police. Ian continued to disclose, and I did report him. It seems that Ian was not traced, and he continues to live at large in the community. I believe he is still a serious threat to children.

> *I enjoy helping [the research] in any way that I can, it's not very often when people want to know or ask about people like me and my desires for children. It's a struggle everyday to be a paedophile and if I helped in any type of way that is great. … twenty years ago I never thought about toddlers or babies in a sexual way but now it's all I can think about and it seems that within the paedophile community if you are attracted to babies that it's more perverse and even the pedo community likes to not make people feel welcome.*
>
> *I am constantly having masturbation fantasies where babies and toddlers are involved, maybe it's because it's so taboo or maybe it's just because that's what I am attracted to. … I have had both gay and straight relationships but was dating a woman that had a daughter that I became very in love with. She was only four years old but I was more in love with her than I was with her mom. … I remember just spending so much time with her whenever I could. One day we were in the pool together and I started to kiss her and started to do things that I was not supposed to do and I felt so guilty about it. Well things continued for another two years until I just could not bring myself to have sex with her mother. I felt like I was acting the whole time and all I would think about during sex was her young daughter. … now I am exclusively attracted to pre-teen children both boys and girls. All the contacts that I have had with children I have never forced them to do anything and when they didn't like anything I would stop and not continue. Yeah maybe I shouldn't have but I did and it's over now.*
>
> *I guess I started to think about toddlers and babies sexually for as long as I can remember but it became well known in my brain that I was sexually attracted to them roughly ten years ago when I dated the woman with the daughter that was four at the time. Her eighteen-month-old cousin was over and her aunt was changing her and I couldn't get my eyes off her beautiful young body. I was amazed by her beautiful vagina and the way that it looked, a few weeks passed and I was changing her the next time they visited that I got so aroused that I started to shake as I was cleaning her. Ever since I have just been hooked on babies and toddlers. They are all that I really think about these days. I mean I still think about older children and all that but it seems that majority of the time when I masturbate it's about babies. … I do think about my sexual attraction to children a lot and it's part of who I am, with a therapist or counsellor I just don't have the funds at this time to pay for one.*

Also I think that certain types of sexual contact hurts children but not all aspects of sex with children is bad, it seems to be a big deal when they are made to feel like victims from their parents and society. I mean yeah intercourse with any child under around fourteen is going to hurt them, but oral sex either way I just don't think is going to harm them or body rubbing or fondling. I mean I think that children around twelve plus can really enjoy intercourse. Some men are not so big in size so I think it's different in all situations. That's just my opinion, yet as a paedophile that only is attracted to children that response is almost expected but that's how I feel.

[At this point, having reminded Ian in my emails of my position as a researcher, I contacted the police and passed on Ian's emails because it was clear that Ian was admitting to criminal actions.]

Something major has happened in my life in the last week or so. I have been outed by a family member as being a paedophile and I have become tired of denying it so I came clean and told my parents that I am in fact a paedophile and that I am exclusively attracted to just children and have no feelings for adults in any sort of way. Of course my parents asked if I have been active with children and I lied yet again and my parents said they would pay for me to go to therapy but I honestly don't feel that I want therapy, I mean what's wrong with being sexually attracted to children? I enjoy getting aroused thinking about them or reading stories and things like that.

Of course I was given an ultimatum about either getting therapy or being banished from family get-togethers and all that because we have dozens of young kids in the family and they don't want a paedophile being around the children and they think it's something you can just turn off and on. Anyway my life is gradually changing and becoming public about the fact that I am a paedophile.

I have been doing a lot of thinking lately and decided to end my relationship with my young boyfriend, it was pretty hard to do but in the end he understood. I have also gradually ended my other sexual relationships with other children that I know. It's crazy how some of them took it but I told them that I will still be their friends and all that and they were cool with that, I just told them that we can't be involved sexually anymore. I guess I have just been caught up in my life of being sexually active with children that I slowly justified it to myself that it's not wrong if the child enjoys the sexual contact but that is not true. Majority of the boys that I have been sexual with have been very into it but that doesn't mean that it's okay to do it. I just feel so comfortable and relaxed with children like I can just be me and maybe in a lot of ways I have the mentality of a young boy and maybe I have some mental problems. I decided to go see a therapist and the main reason is to discuss my paedophilia. Of course I am not going to talk about my actual encounters with children but I am going to talk about my desires and attractions. I just feel like I am like addicted to young children sexually and I don't know what else to do.

I am turning myself in and going to confess and make public all about me and my victims, at first I wasn't going to make it public about the victims but that is what society wants so now they can treat those children like victims even though all of them enjoyed it. I probably won't make it long in prison but that is okay, my life is not that important.

The truth is that no therapist will see me unless I have already been convicted of a child sex crime but I was scared to be honest at first but decided to be upfront and spill the beans and then maybe I could get help. ... I am having a nervous breakdown to be honest with you. With my family's reaction of me being a paedophile to my relationships with boys, my life seems to be on a rollercoaster. My latest relationship that has been going on for a week, I have done something that the boy was not ready for and I feel the only way to make it right is to turn myself in because I really feel bad. In the past I justified my relationships on a sexual level with boys was okay since the boys never said that certain sex acts hurt and none were ever or seemed to be mentally changed by what happened but the last boy that I was with, it went a little too far and he didn't enjoy it like the others and it's a wake-up call to me big-time because I know that I have been lying to myself all these years thinking that it's okay to have sex with young boys when in fact it's really not good at all. I just feel like if I turn myself in that I can stop this reign of terror on boys and stop it all for good. It's like a lust for me that I seem to not have control over and have been struggling with the lust and drive towards boys for the last twenty years and it has to stop now.

I am so scared, I know that paedophiles like myself seem to be and act selfish a lot for our own feelings but I am so scared to go to prison because I know how they treat child molesters and I honestly feel like there is no way that I can help myself or stay alive, they will eat me alive, especially in this day and age. I feel so bad for what I did to the boy and this just is eating me alive and I am feeling such remorse for what I did. As with telling his mother I really don't think that she will even care or comprehend what happened. The boy lives in an area of town that is very poor and he is black and hell even the police don't seem to care about those people in that area and when I met the boy we just clicked and I invited him over to my house and we just became so close. He is such a great kid and things just happened where we had sex and intercourse happened and he just couldn't take it but I kept going because I am a selfish bastard, he is such a sweet boy and I love him very much and since the incident I have had him at my house but we have refrained from intercourse, mostly just foreplay now and I have helped him with the pain.

His mom will just reject him more than she does now, she doesn't give a rat's ass about him. I love the boy and feel like he will just be placed in social services and his life will turn upside down. I just am so confused about what to do. He is such a sweet boy and I want the best for him but I think losing me will just put him in greater danger, he still hugs me when he sees me and I am nervous but he seems to still be relaxed around me and doesn't seem to hate me.

Maybe ending my life will just solve everything.

The other day I was so dead set on turning myself in but now I am confused and I don't want to go to jail. I am also being a chicken-shit about calling Stop It Now because I feel paranoid and all that like somehow they will find out who I am. I know that the only outcome for me in the end is prison and that is not a place that I want to go right now. I am so freaked out right now.

I can't understand how I got myself to this point. I always thought of myself as being a gentle paedophile and now I do something like this to a young boy and I am exactly what I didn't want to become. I have never been able to control my lusts for children and I go around and screw up a boy's life even though he doesn't see it. I spent some time with him last night and we just held each other in bed and it was so awesome. I don't want to lose that bond that we have, he seems to have forgiven me for that night. I also can't come to terms that I am actually a child molester, a sick twisted child molester, hell like my parents said I am a child sex predator. I thought that I was brave enough to do this but it's so hard to do it. I have a nice house, swimming pool, great job and I will lose all of that if I turn myself in and I will also lose my contact with the children that I know. I don't know what to do. … You say that I should turn myself in and that I should be a man about it and do that, yet you know what will happen to me when I go to jail or prison. Child molesters are the lowest of the low and we are treated like shit, yet I should look forward to turning myself in and accepting that fact? You say to contact Stop It Now and all that, well I went to their site and I read the stories and all the offenders served a few months or years in a mental hospital or did a short term in prison but that will not be the case with me because once it hits the public I am sure that boys will be coming out of the woodwork about my sexual relations with them and I will be spending the rest of my life in prison and will never get out, so how am I making myself better if I am going to be in prison or dead?

Well I think it's time for me to be totally upfront and honest with you and of course you will act like you already knew this and that you were just playing along with me because experts like yourself that deal with paedophiles act like that. Yet the honest truth is that I am not active with a young boy or hell any young boys in general, hell I have never ever been active with a child in any type of way. I am a paedophile and that much is true but the difference is that I will never ever be active with a child because I do have morals and I do have ethics. Yet it was all a test to see how you would respond and I want to thank you for the way that you did respond, it showed me that you wanted the best for both parties involved and that's how you came across.

At this point in the correspondence I felt frustrated, angry and very distressed. I did not believe that he had invented the sexual offending. I believed that he was now retracting because he realised the seriousness of what he had said and he was terrified of the impact it would have on his life. I continued to encourage the police to trace his email address and I also continued to encourage Ian to face up to reality. By this point he had obviously decided that he was not prepared to risk his lifestyle for the dubious benefits of potential therapy and the likely punishment for his offences.

I do not know the outcome of this particular case, but what seems clear, even if Ian was in fact exaggerating the extent of his offending behaviour, is that many of the factors that Ian outlines constitute serious barriers to those wishing to seek help for offending behaviour or fears that they may offend in future. Countries vary in the legal requirements placed on therapists to report offending behaviour to the authorities. Countries also vary in the provision of therapists and the availability of state-funded or insurance-funded therapy. As Ian pointed out, state-provided therapy is unlikely to be available until after a person has been convicted of offences, and terror of being reported acts as a barrier to seeking treatment, even though new initiatives such as the telephone and Internet helpline Stop It Now! (at present operating in several countries) can now provide anonymous and confidential advice and support to perpetrators as well as victims.

A final point is that what both the case studies show us is the lack of a strong response by those around the perpetrators. In Fred's case, the police were reluctant and slow to act even when confronted with actual physical evidence showing that Tommy possessed very serious child pornography, and those around Tommy did not challenge him even when he repeatedly struck up close and exclusive relationships with pre-teen girls. In Ian's case, his family apparently accepted his claim that he did not act on his sexual attraction to young children, did not insist he seek help, and did not monitor his behaviour in any way. No one around him apparently challenged his behaviour and he believed, probably rightly, that the local police, whether from racism or for other reasons, would not prosecute him. My own experience was that, having reported him and provided emails where he admitted to sexually abusing children, the case was not followed up. While the rhetoric may be that this society takes child sexual abuse very seriously, the reality all too often lets children down. The concluding chapter of this book suggests some ways forward, so that protection of children may become no longer the hollow sham it all too often is at present.

11 Addressing adult sexual attraction to children

[In my work now] I play daily with children. It gives me the feeling that finally I found what I was created for. And not only the children, I also coach parents, family and teachers. I like this too and it's a great combination. It is as if I understand those children naturally. They feel confident with me. This work gives me a lot of satisfaction. I no longer have strong sexual desire for boys. I think that because of the many contacts there is enough substitution for the specific sexual attraction. ... Maybe you can compare it with a kettle with boiling water in it. If the steam can't get out, the pressure will grow and grow stronger. But if it can get out, there is no problem.

(Oscar)

The way I see it is that I'm hardly unique in the world and there's lot of people like me who have never and certainly will never have any level of sexual contact with children even though we have an attraction to them. If you and I are human beings first and foremost then the only difference between you and me is that I got landed with this as a personal issue and you got landed with it as a social one. People with this attraction have created their own personal safe environment in which children can enter and leave without any danger whatsoever. Speaking to people with personal and practical experience in doing this should surely be the first port of call for society and not people who are sitting in prison as proof only that they couldn't!

(John)

I think your book can make a valuable contribution, because I think paedophiles need to hear these things you've told me, and need to understand that society is a two way street, and that if they want acceptance, they have to commit to behaving appropriately. I've learned this best by being shown tolerance and respect and trust by people I've come out to in real life. I think what's needed is incremental adjustments on both sides. ... so hang in there, please. Say what you believe in your book, but try to give us a voice if you can.

(Tim)

Introduction

This book has been written with the explicit aim of helping all of us in society – children and young people; those with sexual attraction to children and those living with, loving or working with them; and those who simply wish to understand this urgent problem in more depth – to have more information and, having the information, to make better decisions. When I conducted the research on which this book is based, I had four research questions to consider, of which the final question was 'What are the implications of the research findings for improving the level of child protection?' Having set out how the research was conducted and what some of the main findings from the research are, this concluding chapter pulls together the key themes from the research project and presents a new way of thinking about paedophiles and about sexual harm. The implications from this project are relevant to child-protection statutory agencies and charities, to professionals concerned with child protection and children's well-being in a variety of settings, and to adults sexually attracted to children and to all those around them. Some of the material on which these conclusions are based is not presented in this book, but in a companion volume which sets out in much greater detail the cultural milieu within which adult sexual attraction to children is conceptualised and addressed (see Goode, forthcoming).

My research on paedophilia and adult sexual attraction to children has led me to the following three main conclusions.

First, paedophiles exist. This is a scary thought and something many people find difficult to accept. (This refusal to acknowledge reality was shown, for example, in the reactions discussed in the previous chapter, on responses to Tommy and Ian, which made it much harder to ensure that children were effectively protected.) I have been quite astonished, over the last several years, to realise just exactly how difficult it is for people from all walks of life, including professionals and academics, to accept this basic fact that paedophiles do exist and that we know them and often are very fond of them, they live in our communities and are members of our family, our friends, our work colleagues. They are in our churches and other religious settings, they are in positions of authority and trust. Quite often, they may be involved in looking after our children. They may even be involved in child-protection issues. Adults sexually attracted to children probably form something like 2 per cent of the adult male population and no doubt form a relatively high percentage of those adults who choose to work in settings with children and young people. They may well not be exclusively sexually attracted to children; they may form relationships with women, join families, form new families, and parent children. Without getting hysterical about these facts, we need to soberly assess them. How should we respond to this?

My second main conclusion is that policy, media and charity approaches which demonise paedophiles make the situation worse. It may be a good strategy for getting votes, selling newspapers and raising funds to send out messages about 'stranger danger' and portray paedophiles as evil monsters lurking round every corner, but it is not a good strategy for protecting children effectively, which surely should be our most immediate priority. Legislative and bureaucratic responses also are of limited value. The kinds of checks which have recently become law in the UK, which use a database of criminal records to see if an employee or volunteer has a conviction or an allegation relating to child abuse, may indeed assist in keeping some sex offenders out of some posts and I would not argue to rescind such legislation, but on a global level they are unworkable in the impoverished and often chaotic circumstances where the greatest protection is required. Even in highly bureaucratised countries such as the UK, they may be counter-productive in that they promote a false sense of security and a naïve assumption that all known sex offenders will be registered. I reiterate that the purpose of this book is to draw attention to the reality that everyone reading this book is likely to know someone sexually attracted to children. They are also likely to know someone who is sexually abusing children. Those may or may not be the same people. Both practitioners and policy-makers need to pursue methods of child protection which are sensitive, which do not make assumptions, and which focus primarily on what people *do* without being blinded by who they *are*.

Rather than current approaches, we need to learn and apply the lessons from other public health situations. As with HIV, what matters for health protection is not who may or may not have the virus but what actions are performed. Those who are safest are those who assume that anyone may carry HIV and who therefore always follow precautions. In the same way, it matters less, as a general rule, who may or may not be a 'paedophile' pro-vided every organisation always follows careful and rigorous child-protection procedures as a matter of absolute routine.

My third main conclusion is that current criminal-justice interventions do not work. If they did, we would not still have rates of child sexual abuse running at epidemic proportions (Itzin 2006). Criminal justice interventions are a blunt tool. If the only option available is to 'grass' on a perpetrator (who may also be a family member or friend) then many people prefer simply to ignore the abuse and thereby also avoid the shame and embarrassment of the public process of a trial. This means that children are not protected. It also means that, if the only response is punitive, adults who are concerned about their own or a loved one's sexual attraction to children cannot get help and support. They are isolated and often the only source of advice and information they may be able to access is the online paedophile community. In such circumstances, it becomes more likely that the law will be broken and a child will be harmed – or, more typically and tragically, many children over many years. Preventive help needs to be made available.

The lack of help for adults sexually attracted to children is further exacerbated by the lack of knowledge about this area. There is a reluctance to support research to learn more about the experiences of paedophiles or the incidence of sexual attraction to children in the general adult population. Until policy-makers and others find the courage to endorse and commission research in this area, and disseminate relevant findings, child protection agencies are operating with one hand tied behind their backs.

This concluding chapter contains three sections. Section I raises issues about sex and sexuality. It looks at children's sexuality and seeks to explore exactly what it is about adult sexual contact with a child which is so harmful. Section II gives information on four innovative schemes which address adult sexual attraction to children and adult sexual contact with children in a variety of settings, from isolated rural First Nations communities in Canada and Australia to urban settings in the USA, Britain and Ireland. Section III concludes the book and offers a suggested policy for use in organisations working with children and young people.

Section I: Children, sexuality and sexual abuse

In this section I aim to make a few basic points about child and adult sexuality. Anyone who has read this book so far will not be surprised to find that some of my points may be controversial but are also, I hope, grounded in common sense.

My first point is that children below the age of sixteen, the typical legal age of consent around the world, are often interested in sex. The sexuality of children often evokes anxiety for us as parents and within society generally. It also, of course, often evokes anxiety for the developing child too, as they experience their changing body, their new emotions and desires and all the new possibilities of love, fear, failure, pleasure or rejection which go with human sexuality and human romantic relationships. One of the most vocal proponents for the recognition, and valuing, of children's sexuality currently is the American author and journalist Judith Levine, whose book, *Harmful to Minors: The Perils of Protecting Children from Sex,* won the 2002 *Los Angeles Times* Book Prize. Levine's thesis is straightforward: 'sex is not in itself harmful to minors. Rather, the real potential for harm lies in circumstances under which some children and teens have sex...these are the same conditions that set children up to suffer many other miseries' (2002: xxxiii). The socio-economic and cultural circumstances and conditions which Levine identifies as harmful include homophobia, misogyny, dating violence, bigotry, STDs, AIDS, unwanted pregnancy, poverty and racism. She also includes, alongside unwanted pregnancy and sexually transmitted diseases, 'what I'd also consider an unwanted outcome: plain old bad sex' (2002: xxxiii).

Levine's thesis suggests that there is nothing inherently wrong with children under the age of consent being sexually active. For her, it is only the wider social and cultural factors around them which harm them. Levine is writing in a specific social context where the American public is apparently vastly confused – and disturbed – by children and sexuality. She points to recent legal cases and scandals which suggest a shared view 'that physical demonstrations of affection between children are "sex" and that sex between children is always traumatic' (2002: 49). The questions of 'what is normal' and 'what is harmful' when we consider sexual behaviour among children are certainly ones which generate a wide range of answers. Levine generally adopts a *laissez-faire* approach, supporting what she regards as children's right to experiment sexually with one another, and teenagers' rights to have sex with adults. She is not careful to distinguish between children of different ages: in her book they generally all become 'minors', and this elides the distinction between those teenagers aged sixteen years or older who can make informed and knowledgeable choices about sex with people older than themselves and those younger teenagers and children who cannot. That aside, Levine's work is useful in highlighting adult anxiety and confusion over children's sexuality. For example, she points out that when Surgeon General Jocelyn M. Elders suggested masturbation as an appropriate topic for classroom discussion, she was forced to resign. As a society, we seem to be intensely uncomfortable discussing the fact that our children may be sexually curious or may masturbate, even as we allow pornography to become increasingly visible to our children on high-street shelves or television channels, and as we encourage our little daughters to dress in bikinis, thongs and high-heeled shoes and to parade around using the sexualised body language of majorettes or pop stars.

My second point is that children are likely to be sexually exploratory with each other. Common-sense as well as anecdotal evidence, from this study and elsewhere, suggests that children develop sexually at different rates: some children masturbate regularly from a young age, others almost never until they are adult; similarly, some children may start experiencing orgasms while they are still pre-pubertal, others not until they are fully adult. Some children will therefore wish to explore sexual experiences which for other children are beyond their horizon. We can say neither that 'children are asexual' nor that 'children are sexual'. We can only say that children develop sexual curiosity and sexual interest and pleasure at differing rates. Just as the sexuality of women has historically been misrepresented, either discounted altogether in the myth of 'frigid' passivity or else construed as the randy nymphomania so beloved of pornography, so we are in danger of misrepresenting children's experiences. The sexuality which children experience need be neither entirely discounted nor exaggerated. 'Sex play' among children who are broadly at the same developmental stage, which is not coercive and which does not become a guilty, distressing secret, probably helps children resolve their curiosity. It is likely to be brief and episodic, as the child satisfies their curiosity and turns to some other interesting pastime. Sex encompasses a continuum of activities, desires and emotions and, as the child grows into adolescence, the previous 'childish' experiences of giggly 'naughty' looking or touching can provide a reassuring base for more 'grown-up' experiments in kissing, cuddling and consensual exploration. In this, I tend to concur with Levine that 'sex play' (looking, showing, touching, discussing) among children is very unlikely to harm them in any way, provided the child feels able to stop anything she or he does not like and provided the child has learned that her or his body and bodily responses are good, healthy and normal.

My third point is that, if children are sexual and if they are sexually exploratory and curious with other children, it seems – on the face of it – reasonable to suggest that it could be okay for them to be sexually exploratory and curious with adults. What is the harm in sexual contact between children and adults? This is certainly a question which I have been asked repeatedly by paedophiles, with apparently quite genuine sincerity and puzzlement. As a society, we are prepared to acknowledge that 'child sexual abuse' is bad, wrong, immoral and illegal...but why? Each of the three terms, 'child', 'sexual' and 'abuse' have a range of meanings which may cluster about a central point but shade off imperceptibly into other, related terms. When does a 'child' stop being a 'child'? When does a behaviour become 'sexual'? At what point does a behaviour become unambiguously 'abusive'?

When asked to define the harm of 'sexual abuse' we all too often fall back on symptoms, diagnoses, labels, and medical or psychiatric sequalae of 'child sexual abuse' (CSA) as if CSA was some kind of disease or mental illness. All too often, CSA is presented as if it was an attack which the child suffered. Rarely, of course, that may indeed be the case. The child may have been suddenly attacked and overwhelmed by a stranger but far more frequently CSA, like adult rape, is experienced in the context of a relationship and often, like adult rape, in the context of a relationship in which there is or has been trust, love and tenderness. Trying to provide a succinct, workable (and legally intelligible) definition for such a painful and nuanced experience has proved difficult for many. The APA attempts the following:

> There is no universal definition of child sexual abuse. However, a central characteristic of any abuse is the dominant position of an adult that allows him or her to force or coerce a child into sexual activity. Child sexual abuse may include fondling a child's genitals, masturbation, oral-genital contact, digital penetration, and vaginal and anal intercourse. Child sexual abuse is not solely restricted to physical contact; such abuse could include noncontact abuse, such as exposure, voyeurism, and child pornography. Abuse by peers also occurs.
>
> (APA 2001)

By making 'the dominant position of an adult' a 'central characteristic' and then noting that abuse 'by peers' also occurs, the APA signals the conceptual difficulty we are in. In Britain, the main child-protection charity is the National Society for the Prevention of Cruelty to Children (NSPCC), and their definition does lay more emphasis on the relationship aspect of CSA by including 'pressurised, forced or tricked' as part of their definition:

> Sexual abuse is when a child or young person is pressurised, forced or tricked into taking part in any kind of sexual activity with an adult or young person. This can include kissing, touching the young person's genitals or breasts, intercourse or oral sex. Encouraging a child to look at pornographic magazines, videos or sexual acts is also sexual abuse.
>
> (NSPCC 2006)

However, the problem with this definition is implicitly that a judgment must be made on whether there *was* pressure, force or trickery, or indeed 'encouraging'. If a judgment on such ambiguous interactions needs to be made, *whose* judgement would prevail, one wonders. While CSA seems a clear and straightforward concept (an adult forces a child to do something sexual), the term must cover so many potential situations (from violent penetration to kissing; prolonged and repeated physical contact to a fleeting episode of exposure; random aggression from a stranger to sustained sadistic torture by a parent; occurring at birth to age sixteen or older; involving an adult with a baby to two fifteen-year-olds together; sexual murder to mutual exploration) that it becomes attenuated almost to the point of uselessness. And yet, beneath all the confusion and muddle, we are grappling with something which is harmful and which has harmed countless individuals, many of them profoundly. The term 'child sexual abuse' may be a concept, a social construct, but the experience it struggles ineptly to define is very real.

The confusion contained in the term CSA currently works to the benefit of those who wish to argue that adult sexual contact with children (or, as they may prefer to term it, 'child-adult sexual contact', 'age-discrepant relationships' or 'intergenerational intimacy') has the potential to be harmless, or indeed to be positively beneficial (Sandfort 1987; Rind *et al.* 1998; Riegel 2007). This view is at present more muted than it has been, although the journalist Maureen Freely reminds us that radical thinkers in the 1960s and 1970s used to write openly about adult sexual contact with children. For example, Daniel Cohen-Bendit (now a member of the European Parliament) previously wrote about how his 'constant flirt with all the children soon took on erotic characteristics. I could really feel how from the age of five the small girls had already learned to make passes at me...Several times a few children opened the flies of my trousers and started to stroke me...When they insisted, I then stroked them.' Freely also quotes Shulamith Firestone's comment that she hoped, in future, adult relations with children 'would include as much genital sex as they were capable of – probably considerably more than we now believe' (Freely 2001). This attitude to adult sexual contact with children has been voiced in particular by those championing other forms of non-hegemonic sexuality, such as sex between adult men, and an example of this is given by the British gay rights activist Peter Tatchell, who has been involved in the Outrage! campaign and is now active in the Green Party. Tatchell has commented that there are 'many examples of societies where consenting intergenerational sex is considered normal, acceptable, beneficial and enjoyable by old and young alike' (quoted in Bindel 2001). We should not ignore the fact that this opinion continues to be held. As a British citizen, I find it particularly surprising that, even in the twenty-first century, adult sexual contact with children was apparently actively pursued as a cultural practice in at least one British territory – the Pitcairn Islands, a British colony – where it was argued in court that it is 'customary' and culturally normal for adult men to have sex with young girls (Smith-Spark 2004), although ultimately the court did not agree with this view. When we seek to understand CSA, therefore, it is important to recognise that we do so within a continuing, although minority, cultural construction that suggests that in fact children can positively *benefit* from having sex with adults. This is not a position I hold. On the contrary, I argue that, despite its lack of conceptual clarity, the term 'child sexual abuse' points us towards a deep truth which our culture still finds difficulty even in acknowledging and certainly in defining and describing clearly.

In order to be robust, a definition of child sexual abuse (that is, a description of the harm caused by adult sexual contact with children) must be independent of arbitrary historical and cultural contexts; it must not depend on the fact that CSA happens to be defined as illegal within certain jurisdictions, or immoral or unethical within certain systems of thought, or unusual or abnormal within certain social situations. CSA may be all those things, but the harm caused by CSA is independent of those attributes. CSA is generally regarded as illegal, immoral, unethical or wrong *because* it is harmful to the child: it is not harmful to the child solely because it happens in some contexts to be illegal and so on. Even in contexts where there is a cultural consensus that adult sexual contact with children is acceptable, and where no obvious social disapprobation, censure, shame, guilt, punishment or criminal consequence arises from this behaviour, I argue that it remains fundamentally harmful to the child. Proponents of adult sexual contact with children often point to some idealised 'golden age' or 'paradise' when, they argue, sexual behaviour has been or is unproblematically fun and non-exploitative and all is right with the world. Neither those forms of 'relaxed' traditional societies (in which adults, often living in crowded conditions, have sex in front of children and children 'rehearse' sex-play with one another) can provide a 'paradise' of liberated non-puritanical hedonism, nor those forms of 'rigid' traditional societies (in which strictly dichotomised gender roles and kinship-systems and the constraints of family-arranged marriages between often very young women or girls and sometimes substantially older men keep sexuality firmly in check) can give us a 'golden age' of right-thinking sexual control. Both models of society are likely to result in sexual harm. While paedophiles and sexual libertarians in Western cultures often look back to some idealised mythic Other ('Greek love', Polynesia, Papua New Guinea), imagining that, if only they lived there, they would be able to get all the guiltless child sex they could handle, they are deluding themselves. Just as physical chastisement of children is all but universal but remains harmful wherever it is practised, and just as slavery, an institution extending across innumerable civilisations over thousands of years, remains harmful wherever it is practised, so adult sexual contact with children remains harmful regardless of the societal form within which it occurs. Neither traditional nor modern societies have any clear advantage in this regard, and perhaps the most desperate situation is that where traditional societies have broken down in the face of colonialism, racism and socioeconomic destruction. Some paedophiles I have researched find, in societies such as the Northern Territories of Australia, a goldmine of casually available and unpunished sexual use of children, and therefore hold up Aboriginal culture as an example of 'relaxed' sexuality, self-servingly avoiding noticing the epidemic levels of alcoholism, family violence and suicide which also batter these communities.

I also want to make a distinction between 'child sexual abuse' and 'sexual abuse' more generally. 'Sexual abuse' in general permits of the possibility of sexual behaviour which is not abusive. Thus vaginal penetration by a man of a woman could be profoundly abusive or wonderfully pleasurable, depending on how the two people relate to one another. If we rephrase the definition of child sexual abuse by the NSPCC to make it relevant to adults, we could say that 'Sexual abuse is when an adult is pressurised, forced or tricked into taking part in any kind of sexual activity with another adult'. Thus the distinction between 'sex' and 'sexual abuse' is clearly the element of coercion or deceit involved by one adult to obtain sexual gratification from another adult. This is not the case with child sexual abuse. Adult sexual contact with children does not, I argue, require an element of pressure, force or trickery in order to become abusive. It is inherently harmful and remains so even in cases where the child can be regarded as giving 'consent' to the sexual behaviour. (If the sexual contact is also experienced by the child as being pressurised, forced or involving trickery then the harm is magnified, but I am arguing that *the status of being a child* is a necessary and sufficient cause for harm to arise from sexual contact with an adult.)

I am therefore going beyond many current definitions of child sexual abuse here in proposing (1) that CSA is not context-dependent and (2) that CSA does not require an element of coercion. I propose that an understanding of child sexual abuse can be developed which is firmly rooted, not in the vagaries of socio-cultural or legal fashion, but in the biology, neurology and psychology of the developing child. This view of CSA is based on the proposition that there is a fundamental distinction to be drawn between the bodies and minds of children and the bodies and minds of adults, and that this neurophysiological distinction holds true for *Homo sapiens* at any time and in any place, regardless of 'age of consent' laws, child-marriage conventions or other cultural contexts.

The harm involved in adult sexual contact with children therefore depends on the neurophysiological and psychological maturity of the child. As Ruth Kempe and C. Henry Kempe defined it back in 1978, child sexual abuse is 'the involvement of dependent, developmentally immature children and adolescents in sexual activities that they do not fully comprehend, to which they are unable to give informed consent, or that violate the social taboos of family roles' (Kempe and Kempe 1978: 60). The key phrase in this definition is 'developmentally immature'. Whether we wish to term the phenomenon 'abuse', 'assault', 'victimisation', 'contact' or 'intergenerational intimacy', adult sexual contact with children is harmful because of the development processes which the child is still undergoing. Child development is a subject we still have much to learn about. Recent scientific studies are beginning to link together previously disparate aspects within the disciplines of biology, neurology, psychology, and psychoanalysis in order to theorise human development. A science of the emotions is developing, to which psychology, sociology and neuroscience are contributing and which is building an understanding of the links between emotion and cognition, and the ways in which the developing brain of the baby and young child is physically structured according to the psychological environment in which that child grows up (for an accessible overview of these scientific developments, see Gerhardt 2004). In the past fifty years, the physical and social sciences have been able to contribute insights on how closeness and attachment develop between children and those around them (Ainsworth and Bowlby 1965; Bowlby 1988; Stern 2000). These studies have looked at ordinary parenting and also situations where psychological harm is caused. The psychoanalyst Alice Miller, meanwhile, has raised awareness about the harm unintentionally caused by our ordinary everyday habits of parenting and childrearing, such as physical chastisement of children and denial of their emotional responses (Miller 1987, 1995, 2000). These insights go along with developments in international law. Since the League of Nations *Declaration of the Rights of the Child* in 1924, there has been an increasing understanding that children are not small adults, they are humans who are still developing and who therefore require specific protection over and above the protection afforded to other humans. The UN *Universal Declaration of Human Rights,* adopted in 1948, proclaims that the status of childhood is entitled to special care and assistance, and this is reiterated in the UN *Declaration of the Rights of the Child,* in 1959, and the UN *Convention on the Rights of the Child* in 1989. Thus both scientific and legislative advances have emphasised the importance of childhood as a particular moment in an individual's life, when they are not adults, nor are they like adults and should not be treated as adults.

The invisibility of harm related to adult sexual contact with children is related to the invisibility of the concept of autonomy and self-determination for many individuals in traditional societies but especially for the female members of society. As one commentator notes 'In traditional times once a girl's breasts developed she could not remain single' (Bagshaw 2002). This example refers to traditional Aboriginal culture but can be applied all over the world: the lives of girls and women too often have been seen as property to be disposed of as men see fit. In any set-up where men have power over women, a range of harms including sexual harm will occur, whether the situation is one of lawless, anarchic opportunistic sexual violence in the slums and townships, or one of rigid enforced seclusion and control of women within the domestic setting of the traditional village. When men are in charge of a society, the harm caused to women and children is pervasive and extensive (WHO 2009); it is also likely to be unseen, unacknowledged and unaddressed – and without words. All those who care about child protection and human well-being need to recognise that no society or culture is immune: every society, however formulated, contains within it the capacity to abuse, exploit and harm its vulnerable members; at the same time, every society on our planet is now also influenced by mainstream Western culture which has disseminated, alongside an often patchy commitment to democracy and social justice, a view of human sexuality contaminated and degraded by commercial pornography and sexual exploitation.

The psychologist Judith Herman discusses how, given a political context within which to think in new ways, people are able to develop new insights into everyday behaviour. As she says of the beginnings of her own research into the impact of trauma, she slowly learned that:

> It was okay to trust your own observations even if nobody else seemed to think that what you saw made any sense...Even to pay attention to what women say about sex, motherhood, relationships, depends so much on what one thinks a woman ought to be saying, ought to be feeling, is legitimate to express. Unless you have a political movement that says forget what everybody else thinks you *ought* to be feeling, what you *ought* to be saying, get down to it, tell the truth, what did you *actually* think and feel and notice in your body? You need a safe space to be able to do that, you need a political context to be able to do that.
>
> (Herman 2008, interview)

As Herman notes, 'Radical ideas are always very simple, it seems to me. They are only radical because of those [political] obstacles, not because of their complexity.' It was not the intellectual difficulty of understanding the impact of trauma on people which prevented their identification previously; it was the political context which disregarded the individual suffering of certain vulnerable people, primarily women and children. As with 'sexual harassment', 'date rape', 'rape within marriage' and 'child sexual abuse', the theoretical concepts related to complex post-traumatic stress disorder arose initially from consciousness-raising, from women speaking their own lived experiences, theorising the links between personal experience and political context, and naming those experiences for the first time (for further examples of this, see Spender 1980; Armstrong 1996).

From her work, Herman identified complex Post-Traumatic Stress Syndrome (also known as Post-Traumatic Stress Disorder, PTSD), arising from events which instil a feeling of terror and helplessness. Terror is different from fear: under conditions of terror 'some kind of biological rewiring seems to happen' so that even after the danger is over, the person continues to respond both to specific reminders and to generally threatening situations as though the terrifying event were still occurring. The individual experiences flashbacks, nightmares, and also a pervasive sense of numbing, unreality, withdrawal, and possible amnesia to aspects of the event. PTSD varies depending on whether the trauma is repeated and the developmental age at which it first started. It can affect anyone in a situation of 'coercive control'. A specific aspect of PTSD involves 'living in a double reality'. People describe 'simultaneously knowing and not knowing what happened, remembering and not remembering'. People learn to 'divide their consciousness' under conditions of trauma, so that they are no longer clear which is their own and which is the perpetrator's worldview (Herman 2008, interview).

I suggest that the harm caused by adult sexual contact with children is fundamentally related to psychological intrusion and the violation of intimacy. These are aspects which have a correlation with the trauma involved in torture. This is by no means to argue that all sexually abused children are tortured. Rather, it is to identify that what child sexual abuse and torture have in common is the invasive and unbearable intimacy set up in the relationship. This dynamic of overwhelming, coercive intimacy may play itself out even in a context where no harm, and certainly no torture, is intended and where affection and a level of sensitivity and rapport may simultaneously be present. Some adults intend to harm children, or are entirely reckless and indifferent whether they harm them. Some adults who have sexual contact with children genuinely believe that they care about the child. They may feel fond of the child or even feel that they love the child. The abuse may take place in a relationship otherwise characterised by love and trust, for example a parent–child relationship.

How is it possible for the adult not to realise the harm they are causing the child? It is possible because of the structural, social, cultural, interpersonal and psychological processes which underlie every human encounter. These processes produce a situation where the power every adult (even the empathic, liberal, libertarian adult) holds over every child can be rendered invisible. For the child, any capacity to speak their mind freely, even to move freely, is constrained by their inhibition at opposing an adult's will, by their eagerness to please, their desire not to hurt the adult's feeling, their confusion and, fundamentally, their lack of concepts and words to describe their view of the situation. The child is also constrained by their desire not to embarrass the adult or those around them: the child feels protective. More often than we realise, the child may feel compassion for the adult. They may assume responsibility for the situation and for the feelings of the adult. Children are prepared to sacrifice themselves for those they love. Often they would rather take the hurt into themselves, and deny the hurt, than confront the adult or admit to others what is happening.

The processes I have mentioned have properties in common with those which take place during other ambiguous and discordant relationships, where love, hate, despair, abandonment and sacrifice may be painfully interwoven. For example, a child being sexually abused by a teacher and staying silent to protect both the teacher and other adults, including their own parents, is undergoing – to some degree – similar conflicts and decisions to those of an adult (generally a woman) caught up in the relatively brief but destructive dynamics of a 'date rape' or the lengthy and unremitting context of 'domestic violence'. In either case, all too often the abused adult feels ashamed, embarrassed and inhibited from showing anger and distress at what is happening: it is easier to keep quiet, follow the social norms and pretend all is well. In a relationship with an adult which has sexual components, the child may be deeply afraid, but even in situations where the predominant emotions are confusion or embarrassment rather than fear, the processes of socialisation which have taught us 'not to make a fuss' come into play.

Socialisation is an important concept here. It is a shorthand way of understanding some of the structural, social, cultural, interpersonal and psychological processes referred to earlier. If we see the child's experience as occurring at the level of micro-processes (psychological, interpersonal) affecting the situation, then we can bring into focus some of the meso-level (familial, community, cultural) and macro-level (economic, political, social) factors which also bear on the situation.

At the micro-level (which is often where the focus of concern begins and ends), we talk about the 'sequalae' or after-effects of CSA, but the damage has begun before the first sexual contact. For the adult to set up the sexual contact with this child, there is a lack of protectiveness already existing, a lack of safety to speak out, a lack of caring: the child is already isolated and vulnerable. Thus the antecedents to the CSA need healing too. At the micro-level are other factors also which will make it harder for the child to speak out. The child's developmental capacity affects the ability both to make sense of what is going on and set it in a wider context, and also to articulate and express in words what are likely to be highly complex situations and emotions. Overlaid on this developmental difficulty in verbal expression are psychological reactions. Once the child has experienced a sense of invasion through the sexual contact, it becomes harder to break through any existing isolation. Psychologically, it becomes very hard to take anything in when one has been intruded upon. To avoid further intrusion, we may indiscriminately block everything out, including those things (information, affection) which might help us. We may defend against emotional pain and confusion by dissociating. Like a possum 'playing dead' we respond to the disorientating situation (should we approach? Should we avoid?) by simply cutting off, closing down, escaping inwards (Gerhardt 2004). This can make it even harder to speak out, as we literally may hardly speak at all. In the best of circumstances, it is hard for a child to say to an adult, 'Stop. I don't like it.' Even when children do speak up and are heard, their status as a child makes it easy for adults to dismiss or trivialise what they say. It is estimated that conviction rates for CSA remain at fewer than one in fifty, partly because juries and other adults 'still have an inbuilt prejudice that doesn't really take what children say seriously' (Taylor 2004: 17). As well as trivialising children's experiences generally, adults, including professionals such as police officers or social workers, may want to block out what the child says because it is too painful, especially if they themselves were abused as children or now have children of the same age. It can be easier to ignore than to recognise 'This could be me. This could be my child'. All these factors contribute to the CSA happening in the first place, continuing undetected and unpunished, and harming the child by invalidating what she or he tries to express about their feelings.

At the meso or cultural level, many factors come into play. For example, there is still a view that sex is unproblematically good and that resistance to sex must be related to 'prudery' or 'inhibitions'. Older and more powerful individuals may have a genuine sense of wishing to initiate or liberate someone younger into sexual experience, and regard any opposition as mere ignorant reluctance to be overcome by persuasion or force 'for your own good'. They may believe that this is not harmful, that the child or young person 'will thank me in the end'. Cultural standards which position men as powerful, authoritative, decisive and dynamic encourage such an attitude of breaking through resistance. Again, we can see analogies with 'date rape'. At the same time, almost universally, men are not encouraged to be sensitive to emotional cues. While little girls may have been spending their childhood talking with their friends and picking up the social skills to develop 'woman's intuition', little boys are more likely to have experienced playground fights and bullying that left them licking their wounds and developing a carapace to protect against recognising emotions – other people's or their own. Not only men but women too may find it hard to pay attention to emotions, and to those of children especially. Children who are in psychic pain trigger very powerful responses in the adults around them. It takes emotional maturity to psychologically hold or 'contain' the child's pain and help them manage it. It is much easier to brush it aside ('Don't be silly, of course it doesn't hurt') and thereby to avoid feeling our own pain as well as the child's, or else to quickly indulge what we believe is the child's immediate need at that time ('There, there. This will make it better. Now you're fine, so stop fussing.'), without pausing to engage with and really hear that individual child's own unique needs. It is so easy to give a child what *we* think they need. There are often family or community-specific child-rearing traditions which reinforce these cultural assumptions that children can be ignored, with their needs either brushed off or covered over, but not heard. In such a context, even when the child has been able to speak up, it is hard for an adult to hear, and take seriously, a child saying, 'Stop. I don't like it'.

At the macro-level, too, there are many factors which contribute to CSA, enable its continuation and exacerbate the harm. Women or adolescents who sexually abuse children may be socially invisible, and this is true also for those who have not yet offended but are concerned that they might. Meanwhile, socialisation makes it less likely that any man concerned about his actions will be open in seeking help: it is a cliché that a man will not even stop the car to ask for directions and that asking for help in any circumstances is seen as not a masculine trait (Gray 1992). Seeking counselling or therapy for difficult situations, especially when they involve one's sexuality and especially when they involve deviant sexuality which can lead to illegal behaviour, becomes increasingly remote as a possibility. Men would rather commit suicide than admit to feelings of depression or hopelessness: in Britain, for example, three times more men than women commit suicide and it is the most common cause of death in men under the age of thirty-five (Samaritans 2004;

Department of Health 2005). Societies reinforce this response by not providing help to prevent offending and by setting up punitive strategies instead, against which a 'real man' may be tempted to rebel. A free-thinking, free-wheeling outlaw may be a more congenial identity for some men than a despairing 'failure' who has to admit to the need for help. Thus, in a context in which it is hard for a child to say, and for an adult to hear, 'Stop. I don't like it', it is also hard for the adult to say, 'I need help.'

Ultimately, all these processes of socialisation, and many more, surround the adult and the child and provide the pernicious context within which the psychological harm to the child's sexual integrity goes unnoticed and unacknowledged. It is not surprising, perhaps, that abusing adults genuinely do not seem to understand the harm that they are causing. Fran Henry, the founder of Stop It Now!, was sexually abused by her father from the age of twelve to sixteen. As she describes it, when she confronted him later:

> I found my father did not understand how much damage he did to me when he abused me. ... Ignorance, not evil, lies at the heart of this devastation wrought on us and on our sexuality. Ignorance and a good measure of human greed and fear. As I witnessed my father's ignorance, I realised that he was caught in a great trap of how society dealt with sexuality and sexual abuse – through silence and evasion.
>
> (Henry 2005: 4–5)

When an adult has sexual contact with a child, no matter how much the adult may regard the relationship as loving, it is harmful. It coerces the child into something which is invasive and intrusive, an intimacy which the child has as yet no developmental boundaries to protect against. The younger the child, and the more intimate the context, the more fundamental is the distortion of the child's developmental experiences. The child's autonomy and self-determination are violated; the need to explore and learn about one's own sexual being at one's own pace, under one's own control. The child's first experience of a sexual relationship becomes a coerced experience, deeply embedded and re-experienced within the child's body and mind. The worldview of the adult becomes incorporated into the worldview of the child as a confusing and inarticulate 'double reality'. The psychological sense of one's own body as inviolable, under one's own control, for one's own self, is broken. Fran Henry talks of a new precept of sexual integrity to heal us from sex repressed or sex too expressed, from ignorance or abuse. She suggests that, within a context of sexual integrity:

> Perhaps we could then see our attraction to the physical beings of children, how by their nature they draw us in. At times we might even feel sexual or erotic feelings ourselves in response to them. With sexual integrity we would understand and appreciate the pleasure they show us and we would not be embarrassed to admit to ourselves or to others our feelings. We

could also see that people who sexually abuse children rob them not of innocence to their sexual natures, but their chance to discover and integrate sexual unfolding on their own terms.

(Henry 2005: 10)

In this section, I have suggested that children are often sexually interested and sexually exploratory. I have looked at the difficulty of defining 'child sexual abuse' and the fact that there is still a minority view that adult sexual contact with children can be harmless or positively beneficial for children. I have argued, however, that it is the distinctive developmental status of being a child which makes sexual contact with an adult harmful and, as we learn more about human emotional and cognitive development and more about how humans respond to trauma, we become increasingly sensitised to understanding the complex ways in which adult sexual contact with children is harmful, not necessarily obviously but profoundly, through an intimate psychological invasion which children do not have the ability to fend off. The following sections explore initiatives and suggested policies for preventing and reducing child sexual abuse.

Section II: New initiatives in addressing adult sexual attraction to children

As noted in the Introduction, it is increasingly becoming recognised that criminal justice interventions, on their own, are a blunt tool. Fortunately, there are more radical approaches to child protection now being developed around the world. Building on principles of restitutive or restorative rather than retributive justice, and distinct from a traditional, centralised and formalised top-down reliance on professional intervention and surveillance, these new initiatives tend to be local, small-scale, informal, imaginative, and fired by a desire for political change as well as individual and community responsibility. They include, for example, Stop It Now!; Circles of Support and Accountability; Hollow Water; and B4U-ACT. All of these have in common that they locate sexual abusers and paedophiles in their everyday environment – their local community.

The Stop It Now! campaign was started by Fran Henry in 1992 in the USA and is now also operating in Britain and Northern Ireland. It is based on Fran's own experience as a survivor and her tremendous courage in publicly discussing the complexity of being abused by someone you know and love – and continue to know and love. As she says of her father who abused her, 'I could tell you...stories that would make you hate him in an instant. But at the next moment I could tell you stories of his humanity, his strength and his history that might leave you wanting to admire him. Complex, isn't it?' (Henry 2001).

Her courage in not reducing her father to a one-dimensional cardboard cut-out of a hate figure, a straw-man paedophile, means that she can propose ways forward to protect children. She has based the work of Stop It Now! on three simple principles. The first is to talk openly about sexual abuse, without shame, as we would talk about drink-driving or cancer or any other public-health issue. The second is to hold abusers accountable, at the same time as understanding them as human beings. The third is to focus on prevention by strategies such as awareness-raising and sex education for the general public, together with effective treatment including voluntary treatment and work with abusers, their partners and their families. As mentioned in the preceding section, Henry's focus is on sexual integrity, the enjoyment of pleasurable and consensual sexuality, and the aim of the campaign is to increase sexual knowledge and reduce ignorance and shame. Stop It Now! run public-education campaigns and helplines, and have leaflets and other material available, providing straightforward information and advice.

Circles of Support and Accountability (known simply as Circles) is a Canadian initiative established by a Mennonite Church pastor, Harry Nigh, in Toronto in 1994, which has also now begun to be used in Britain. Like Stop It Now!, this example shifts the balance of responsibility away from professionals back to the local community and is based on the premise of the community taking responsibility for protecting itself. It is more narrowly focused on the treatment of abusers, and in particular relapse prevention, but again adopts a community-based, public health approach which avoids demonising paedophiles and child sexual abusers. On release from prison, a convicted sex offender is resettled into the community with the help of six trained volunteer supporters, who each commit to spend time with the offender one day per week, and who all get together with him (I am not aware that any women offenders have been involved as yet) as a group on the seventh day. The goal is to support the offender daily, and to hold him accountable for his actions. As members of Circles explain:

> It's all about people forming and creating community, and not excluding anyone. It's about looking at people as people. ... The key thing is the acceptance of that individual as a member of society – a contributing member – not as a paedophile, who has only and will only ever have that label. If you don't let them forget that, then that's all they will ever be – a paedophile.
>
> (quoted in Silverman and Wilson 2002: 178)

The emphasis on community contrasts strongly with many of the quotations on the lack of support experienced by respondents in the MAA Daily Lives research project, and with this comment by Dan Markussen, a spokesperson for the Danish Paedophile Association, on the loneliness and lack of community which paedophiles in general are likely to feel, whether they are convicted offenders or not: 'Most pedophiles lead a terrible life. They can't tell anybody about their feelings. They have to fake interest in adults. Many live in social isolation which leads to weirdness' (quoted in Flanagan 2004). Perhaps, in the future, initiatives such as Circles can be set up to support paedophiles to live law-abiding lives as a preventive process, *before* they have already broken the law and harmed children.

The third example of an innovative response is from Hollow Water, an isolated rural indigenous community of approximately 1,000 people in Manitoba, Canada. Here, a carefully worked-out form of community engagement, known as 'community holistic circle healing' (CHCH), has been set up. This has been cited as an example of good practice in *Ampe Akelyernemane Meke Mekarle: 'Little Children are Sacred'*) (Wild and Anderson 2007), a report addressing the endemic child sexual abuse currently experienced in Aboriginal communities in the Northern Territory, Australia. The *'Little Children are Sacred'* Report notes that concepts of justice among indigenous peoples are different from more mainstream approaches (Wild and Anderson 2007: 132–3), but it would appear that any community might benefit from considering such an holistic approach to justice and healing. In whatever context, it seems self-evident that an integral part of any protective measure needs to include community-based initiatives. Such initiatives reinforce ordinary, everyday, human interactions and individual responsibility and hold us all accountable – to our families and our wider communities – for all our actions. A member of Hollow Water CHCH, Berma Bushie, has described this process, which has similarities to Circles of Support and Accountability but with a much greater emphasis on the integration of the whole community.

> In 1984 a Resource Team was formed to work on healing and development. ... The first disclosure of sexual abuse came in 1986. Before that time, no one talked about it. ... At that point there was no turning back. It became very clear that there had been a great deal of sexual abuse going on for many years, but that talking about it was taboo. ... [As healing occurred, there] was a dramatic increase in the number of sexual abuse disclosures. The Resource Team soon realised that there was a fundamental conflict between what the justice system does with offenders and what the community needed to do. ...
>
> 1. [There is] an initial investigation to find out what really happened. The victim's story is gently and lovingly recorded. The victim's safety and, as well, the presence of reliable and trusted people to support the victim through the crisis is ensured.
> 2. Once it has been determined (beyond reasonable doubt) that abuse has taken place, the abuser is confronted and charged. At this stage, the combined power of the law and the community are used to force the abuser to break through his or her own denial to admit to the abuse, and to agree to participate in a healing process. The abuser's choices are a) to plead guilty and then to be sentenced to probation requiring full cooperation with the healing process, or b) to be abandoned to the courts, with jail as the probable outcome.

3. If the abuser agrees to the healing road, he or she then begins a three to five year journey, which ends in restitution and reconciliation between the abuser and the victim, the victim's family and the whole community. When an abuser commits him or herself to the healing process, the CHCH team asks the court for a minimum of four months to assess the authenticity of the commitment. ... During the four-month period, abusers are asked to undergo a process of looking deeply into themselves and really breaking through the denial to admit to themselves and others what they have done and how their actions have hurt others. This process involves four circles.

(Bushie, n.d.)

As Bushie describes it, this process is in no way a soft option. Working in the circles is challenging and slow. Initially, in the first series of circles the person is asked to share what they have done with the circle and with a sexual-abuse counsellor and sometimes other professionals as well. This is a difficult process, and at first the abuser can only describe the offence vaguely. As they feel the love and support of the circle, they are gradually able to admit everything. During this stage, the abuser must be willing to fully engage in the healing process and, as they do, the circle works to help the abuser become a healthy and productive member of the community. The second circle requires the abuser to involve their family. The abuser must admit to their partner and children what they have done, and deal with the family's response. The third circle repeats this process with the abuser's wider family: their own parents, grandparents and other family members. The fourth circle is the sentencing circle. Bushie explains that, in this circle, abusers must tell the whole community (represented by whoever attends the circle) what they have done and what steps they have already taken on their healing journey.

At the same time as working with the abuser, the community holistic circle healing process also works with the victim and with any family members or others who are in need of support. Each case of abuse may therefore result in eight or more people being involved. This is an intensive process of healing and reintegration, which does not duck away from accountability and an emphasis on the ownership of the abuse by the abuser. Its strength lies in the way it brings the legal system 'into the circle of the community in order to creatively use that system to help heal the community' (Bushie, n.d.).

The fourth example, B4U-Act, differs from the previous three examples in that it explicitly includes self-defined paedophiles as part of the team. Set up in 2003 in Maryland in the USA, B4U-Act is slowly developing a profile. As it notes on its website, b4uact.org (July 2008), it is

a unique collaborative effort between minor-attracted people and mental health professionals to promote communication and understanding between the two groups. Our goal is unique and unprecedented: to make effective and compassionate mental health care available to individuals who self-identify as minor-attracted and who are seeking assistance in dealing with issues in their lives that are challenging to them. We want to give them hope for productive and fulfilling lives, rather than waiting for a crisis to occur.

B4U-Act is also associated with another initiative, Lifeline, which is an online counselling and befriending service using a real-time chat facility. Lifeline has worked with suicidal people and appears, from comments by respondents on MAA Daily Lives Project, to provide a significant and valued source of support. Lifeline is advertised through the major pro-paedophile websites and has been running for around seven years. Like B4U-Act, Lifeline is organised by volunteers who include self-defined paedophiles. Neither B4U-Act nor Lifeline appears explicitly to promote a child protection model or explicitly to advocate abstaining from sexual contact with children. For example, in discussion with the founder of Lifeline, it was stated:

> *It is possible for people to develop a positive identity as a paedophile/child-lover/MAA and so on, which does not include within it any sexual contact with a child. It probably goes without saying that the move towards non-sexual contact in these times results from the harsher penalties put in place legally. … At Lifeline we don't advocate visitors choosing any certain life-style. It is not part of our mission to steer visitors away from sexual rela-tionships with children. In our community, due to the illegal ramifications of sexual relationships between adults and minors, there is little talk about sexual relationships. We aren't allowed to discuss the issue because it's been made illegal for us to do so.*
>
> (Personal email correspondence, 12 February 2008)

In distinction to the previous examples, there is no community engagement other than with mental health professionals, and there is no sense of restitutive or restorative justice for those who have harmed children. The emphasis is on providing paedophiles with friendship, support and access to mental healthcare, although it is recognised that:

> Forcing minor-attracted people to remain secretive and without access to mental health care does not protect children. Stigmatising and stereotyping minor-attracted people inflames the fears of minor-attracted people, mental health professionals, and the public, without contributing to an understanding of minor-attracted people or the issue of child sexual abuse. Minor-attracted people are unable to seek services when they want them, and mental health professionals are unable to reach out to them. Perpetuating secrecy, stigma, and fear can lead to hopelessness and even self-destructive or abusive behavior on the part of minor-attracted people, and disrupts the fabric of society. It is also important to realise that some of the children or adolescents in need of protection are themselves developing an attraction to children.
>
> (B4U-Act, FAQ, updated 31 August 2008)

Despite their differences, what all these approaches do have in common is a rejection of heavy-handed, legalistic and over-bureaucratised systems in favour of more imaginative responses emphasising personal responsibility and face-to-face communication. The approaches given here view paedophilia and the sexual abuse of children as complex human experiences which take place within relationships and communities, and which are the outcomes of an irreducibly intricate mix of beliefs, understandings, histories, fantasies and desires. Whether the focus is on healing the harm caused by sexual abuse, or working to prevent that harm from occurring in the first place, the main message for practitioners and policy-makers is that ultimately the key to child protection lies less with the formalised bureaucratic processes of law than with 'forming and creating community, and not excluding anyone'.

Section III: Keeping children safe

As we emerge into the twenty-first century, we are frightened and dazed by conflicts and threats. The theme of much work in contemporary sociology and cultural theory is of risk, fragility and despair, speaking of our sense of fear and hopelessness as we seek to understand – if no longer to control – global dangers. The great project of the Enlightenment, the striving of a whole civilisation towards rationality, scientific discovery and upward progress now seems doomed, fractured by internal dissent and by social, political, economic and environmental forces we had believed were long overcome. News of phenomena seemingly from hundreds of years in the past – plagues, crusades, child-brides, punishment by flogging, death by stoning, piracy on the high seas – arrive incongruously through RSS feeds onto our Blackberries and iPhones. In the midst of this disorientation, people speak of 'compassion fatigue' as we view, yet again, endless parades of wizened, starving baby-faces on our television screens and hear incomprehensible figures for the numbers of AIDS orphans, the numbers of deaths by drought, by famine, by war, by earthquake, by flood, by tsunami...

In this context, how do we respond to children who need protection? The historian Carolyn Dean, in a discussion on the fragility of empathy, argues that the 'possibility that there is a continuity between a "normal" person and a monstrous one and that indeed that person may be lurking anywhere and may even be "us" was first rendered thinkable and discussable after the Holocaust' (2004: 136). We live post-Holocaust, in a time when people alive today experienced mass murder bureaucratically organised and carried out under the impassive gaze of innumerable citizens. We struggle to make sense of the numbness, the indifference and, now, the 'pornographic' re-presentations of such cruelty and violence. We have largely forgotten, meanwhile, other massacres of millions of civilians carried out by Pol Pot, Stalin, Mao Zedong and other tyrants. We live in a time when a resurgence of traditional practices such as female genital mutilation, 'honour killings', polygamy and the trafficking and trading of human beings takes places against the incongruous backdrop of an increasing emphasis on international human rights. Highly paid human-rights lawyers meticulously defend the freedoms of their wealthy clients, while no doubt their toilets are cleaned by illegal immigrant labourers existing without access to even basic rights. Global human society is exploding, and the fragments are fracturing away from each other at an unprecedented pace. Despite international movements for democracy, a quarter of all countries in the developing world still have laws impeding women owning land or homes (UN Human Settlements Programme 2003): this fundamental legislative, economic, social and cultural disparity prevents women having equal power in protecting their children.

Meanwhile, in the developed world, child protection is frequently viewed as little more than a bureaucratic process. The response of governments in the UK, the USA, Australia and other countries in the past few years has been to increase the capacity of the police to identify and monitor offenders and to 'vet' and 'bar' known offenders from occupations involving children, by using databases such as ViSOR (the Violent and Sex Offenders Register). This is an approach which could be seen as analogous to the War on Terror, an attempt to seek out a hidden but well-defined threat and render it harmless before damage is done. This approach relies on sophisticated and expensive tools of information-gathering, surveillance and registration and it springs from the same simplistic and reductive worldview which sees identity cards as making us safer in the fight against terror. Such an approach is partial and inade-quate. Like the War on Terror, the fight is, in reality, not so much against an isolated and extremist few (those who attack and murder) but for the hearts and minds of wider segments of society. It will always be only a small minority of sexual abusers who are known to the authorities: therefore any child-protection strategy which relies on bureaucratic processes of monitoring, surveillance and registration to vet and bar offenders from working with children will always be largely unsuccessful. Even where those who are merely suspected, as well as those who are actually convicted, are included on offender data-bases this will continue to represent only a tiny proportion of all the people who have or who are currently sexually abusing children, or who have the desire and intention to sexually abuse in the future.

At the end of this book, the view is bleak. Paedophiles are not evil monsters out there, waiting to pounce on our children the moment we relax our vigilance: no, paedophiles cannot be excised from our culture, there is no clean 'surgical strike' which can hit them, there is no separation between them and us. Instead, we are all entangled together, the abusers with the abused, the inno-cent with the complicit. Superficially, this may appear a similar point to Kinsey's: sex offending, he argued, is a statistical norm and therefore, in the words of his biographer Jonathan Gathorne-Hardy, 'everybody's sin is no sin at all'. My conclusion is different. Wife-beating too has been, over the gen-erations, statistically normal: capital punishment, corporal punishment of children, child labour, slavery – all have, for almost all of human history, been statistically normal. Everybody's sin (our indifference, our abuse of children) remains a sin. But there are cultural shifts which take seriously the rights of women and children. The fact that a book such as this can be written suggests that changes may be occurring.

I will end this book with advice emanating from a surprising source. Dr Parker Rossman, an ordained clergyman, published a book in 1976 with the depressing title *Sexual Experience between Men and Boys*. The book in general contains the kind of self-serving hooey one might expect with such a title. However, it ends with some practical recommendations which are both sensible and humane, and which I have adapted in the following suggestions.

Provide therapy

The first recommendation by Rossman is to increase the level of therapy available, especially to younger people. Adolescents are the ones most likely to be beginning to feel 'different' and concerned about their sexual attraction to children; their attraction will be starting to become obvious to them as they and their peers move away in age from childhood playmates. It is at this point that sensitive and caring counselling will be of most value. It will reduce the suffering of the adolescent himself, and will provide a better outlook for his well-being in future and his ability to manage his sexual attraction throughout his lifetime, while staying within the law. I would add to this the possibility of allowing those adults who are sexually attracted to children access to masturbation material which is not based on images of actual children but which is, for example, graphic cartoons such as lolicon manga. If our priority is to protect children, then perhaps some sexual outlet needs to be provided, but one which avoids illegality and which does not involve harm to any child. In the same way that methadone maintenance therapy is designed to reduce the black market in opiates, policy-makers might courageously examine the option of reducing demand for illegal material by supplying, or permitting, substitute masturbation material for those who are clear that their primary erotic attraction is to children.

Equip children and teenagers to cope

This recommendation is far from any simplistic 'just say no' campaign which puts the onus (and implicitly the blame) on children to protect themselves individually. This recommendation is about young people working together as a group to protect one another. As Rossman suggests, 'No youngster is as safe from sexual molesting as when he is with a group of self-disciplined, well-informed peers, who as a group are in control of their own situation. Youngsters can and will protect each other from strangers and outsiders' (1976: 219). Rossman is thinking here of adolescent boys at risk from predatory paedophiles but the concept of children banding together and dispelling the fear, isolation and stigma of sexual threat from adults is an empowering one. I would suggest that the more children are encouraged to talk openly about sexual issues, the less likely they are to stay silent when threatened with a unpleasant situation, whether from a stranger or within the family. It is silence and isolation which enable sexual abuse to exist, so the ability and confidence to tell others – and possibly even band together to confront the abuser – may provide one of the best antidotes to vulnerability. In order to equip children and teenagers to cope, it is also useful for them – and the adults around them – to be aware of warning signs that someone may have a problem with sexual interest in children, and to develop a Safety Plan. Lists of warning signs and a useful Family Safety Plan are available from Stop It Now!, and can be accessed at www.stopitnow.com/warnings.html.

Change the supporting structures

The relevance of this recommendation will vary with the context, but Rossman suggests offering employment or other options for adolescent boys to reduce the likelihood that they will find excitement and rewards only in delinquency, drugs and sexual relationships with pederasts. His main point is that, 'Adults who wish to oppose pederasty must volunteer their own time and money to assist the social agencies, and not merely rely upon passing laws to punish the victims of their previous neglect' (1976: 221).

Part of spending time with young people must include affectionate physical contact. Rossman noted earlier (1976: 148) that 'youngsters seek physical reassurance and affection [from paedophiles] in young adolescence when they are at a stage of life when no one else is hugging them any more.' I suggest that increased displays of physical affection make sexual abuse *less* likely, because the young people are getting the warmth and physical contact our bodies crave and also because some paedophiles will find it easier to resist sexual temptation when they are able to express care and closeness and thus meet their psychological if not their sexual needs. Policies which rigidly and absurdly forbid any physical contact between adults and children make it difficult for children (and adults) to know what is appropriate touch. As Judith Levine (2002) has commented, children need to be able to say 'yes' as well as 'no', and shoulder touches, hand-holding and hugs from trustworthy adult friends should ideally be part of all children's experiences.

Face up to adult sexual attraction to children

This final recommendation from Rossman is very much in line with the message of this whole book, and with other initiatives such as Stop It Now!'s public-health and public-education approach to child sexual abuse. Rossman suggests that staff manuals should contain helpful comments such as that 'good, well-intentioned men sometimes succumb to sexual temptation with boys without intending it', making it possible for staff and volunteers to express their concerns without being stigmatised, and so to receive timely help in resisting temptation and keeping children safe.

Rossman provides an example of a six-point staff policy statement which could provide the basis for a policy to be adopted in any organisation where adults come into contact with children. The following suggested Policy Statement offered here is an adaptation based on the policy provided in full in Rossman (1976: 222–4). It is adapted to reflect new legislation, for example in the UK, which requires checking of criminal records for any post involving working with children or vulnerable adults. It is also adapted to make it relevant to any adult sexually attracted to any child (rather than simply men attracted to boys) and it has a greater emphasis on child protection and emotional responses than the original version.

I would support using written policy to encourage an atmosphere where clear boundaries are understood, adhered to and openly discussed, and where sexual attraction can be acknowledged without panic and without complicity. Such a policy might, for example, sit alongside a Code of Conduct which would set out in clear terms what is acceptable as well as what is not acceptable (for example, giving and receiving hugs but not for a child to sit on an adult's lap; being alone with a child with the door open but not with the door closed) and which would also set out more details on the procedure should the Code of Conduct be broken. Clear statements, written in common-sense terms, enable both adults and children to know the boundaries while still retaining spontaneity and warmth in their dealings with one another. It seems to me that such an atmosphere would be likely to result in a far safer environment for children than the current typical situation which relies only on bureaucratic processes of legislative disclosure and where everyone feels far too embarrassed or stigmatised to express concerns or to ask for help.

Suggested policy statement for organisations working with children or adolescents

(A)   Every new staff and volunteer member (in addition to having an interview, references and a criminal-records check, where this is the national policy or is advised) will be informed, at the time of employment and periodically thereafter, that many adults (predominantly men) are not aware of their own capacity to be sexually aroused by children, including the capacity of ordinarily heterosexual men to find themselves sexually attracted to boys. It will be explained that this attraction does happen at times and that there is help available. At the same time, it will be made clear that the organisation will not tolerate sexual contact between adults and children. New staff will be informed that if they find themselves so tempted there are confidential counselling resources available to them, at no cost, to help them understand and handle any problem which might arise.

(B)   Senior and more experienced staff will be given staff training to help them recognise warning signs and types of behaviour which indicate that an adult may be sexually interested in a child. They will also be given training on how to raise the subject initially and how to provide a friendly and confidential warning, along with the offer of counselling and help. All staff must feel encouraged to discuss this topic and the balance between confidentiality and accountability to line-managers must be clear.

(C)   Where there is reliable evidence that an adult has *sought* (but not engaged in) any type of sexual activity with a child, the adult is to be warned by senior staff that a repetition of such behaviour could lead to arrest. If the staff member chooses to resign, concerns will be passed on to relevant authorities. Otherwise, the staff member must enter into a programme of counselling and therapy under the super-vision of senior staff. The organisation will operate on the policy that someone who has such temptations and is aware of them is a better risk than someone who has such temptations and is not yet conscious of them. Open and honest acknowledgement and support not to offend are a better method of risk-management than secrecy and denial. Some adults who choose to work with children may do so because of, not despite, the fact that they find children sexually attractive. Such adults may have great love and commitment to offer their work and this can be supported and valued, provided clear boundaries are in place, and provided they are receiving counselling to address their sexual thoughts about children.

(D)   Where there is reliable evidence that an adult has been involved in any type of sexual activity with any child (including use of child porno-graphy or child sex tourism), then the staff member will be dismissed and details will be passed to the police. The child or children involved, if they are within the organisation, will be counselled and comforted on the basis that they, as minors, are not responsible for any sexual behaviour by an adult or for any consequences such as that adult losing their job: these consequences are the result of criminal beha-viour which the adult chose to do. Children (and affected staff) will be counselled to deal with their feelings which may include anger, sad-ness, loss, confusion, embarrassment, blame, guilt or a sense of betrayal. Parents will also be informed and offered support. Where a court-case takes place, children, their parents and staff will be sup-ported through the process by senior members and the counselling team. The policy of the organisation will be to avoid dramatising or minimising the situation but to concentrate on dealing sensitively with emotional responses in a timely manner.

(E)   It is fully recognised and accepted by the organisation that children are sexually interested and experimental, particularly as they move into adolescence. Staff will make it clear to all children involved with the organisation that a whole range of sexual and romantic feelings are to be expected, that managing one's own sexual interest and sexual arousal is all part of growing up, and that any concerns about any aspect of sex or sexuality can be discussed at any time with staff or the counselling team. At the same time, 'sex play' is inappropriate at organisational activities and sexual harassment or molesting by anyone towards anyone else will not be tolerated. It is important for children as well as staff to feel comfortable with everyday physical contact, and ordinary physical affection and contact between staff and children is encouraged. Sex education and child protection leaflets such as that provided by Stop It Now! or children's charities may be appropriate to supplement these messages. Staff will also be given training regarding healthy sexual development and behaviours in children.

(F)   If a child develops an emotional, romantic or sexual 'crush' on a staff member, this will be discussed at staff meetings and handled sensitively to avoid rejection or hurt and to make the experience a growing, maturing one for the child. If a staff member develops a 'crush' on any child or adolescent, this will similarly not be hushed up or treated as a taboo situation but calmly recognised and addressed, keeping child protection as the priority. Adults will be expected to manage and control their feelings in a mature and responsible manner, with counselling as appropriate. Healthy, open, supportive friendships between children and adults can be good for all concerned, but the organisation will not tolerate secrecy or favouritism.

(G)   If an adolescent is observed developing sexual interests in younger children, this should be taken seriously but calmly. The adolescent should be given counselling and insights to help understand society's expectations and to develop necessary sexual self-control. Staff (and children) might benefit from sources of advice such as the Stop It Now! booklet 'Do Children Sexually Abuse Other Children?' in order to understand this situation. The policy is to help the adolescent to feel understood, accepted and supported in managing their feelings and controlling their behaviour, so that they grow up into a responsible and loving adult.

As a mother, an organisational policy such as this would make me feel that my children were better protected here than in an organisation with no written policy and no recognition of the problem. I would also feel that my children stood a better chance of protection here than in any organisation holding what seem to be the usual unrealistic assumptions: that no paedophiles work there or could ever work there; that no child sexual abuse could ever take place; that all 'bad apples' are screened out; and that if any incidents were to occur they must either be treated as an unprecedentedly wicked and scandalous crisis...or simply covered up.

The whole intention of this book has been to enable us, as a society, to understand that adult sexual attraction to children does exist and that the best way to address it is through awareness, empathy and clear boundaries, by accepting that the way to protect children is to allow us all to talk openly about our feelings, no matter what they are, while holding ourselves responsible for our actions, no matter what they are.

> For every complex problem, there is a simple answer, and it's wrong.
>
> (Internet saying)

The author would be pleased to hear from you if you have any comments in relation to this book. She can be contacted at Sarah.Goode@winchester.ac.uk or via the publishers.

Please note that there may be further editions of this book, or further publications to arise from this work. Any correspondence which you choose to send may be used as data and may be published. If you disclose details of previously unreported criminal activity and you are identifiable, the information will be passed on to the relevant authorities. Otherwise, full anonymity and confidentiality will be respected for any comments or insights you may wish to share.

Appendices

The logo for this project was kindly designed and provided by an individual in collaboration with the 'participant coordinators group'. The logo was made available to me in anticipation of the original data collection project, using focus groups in the USA, which was intended to be conducted during July 2006. It was only when this did not happen that the online questionnaire survey was developed and conducted. The logo was used on the website set up by the 'participant coordinators group' to promote this project, where details of the project and downloadable copies of the Information Sheet and Questionnaire were made available.

Please note that, as the research methodology was based on grounded theory, the questions and form of wording evolved over the period of data collection in accordance with data and feedback received from respondents. The wording of the Information Sheet was agreed with the Ethics Committee and remained the same throughout the course of the research (although the contact details provided for me were removed on some versions, in compliance with a request from the 'participant coordinators group', who were concerned about my safety.) The Questionnaire, however, was continually revised and refined over the course of the research, although the changes tended to be very minor. I added a few additional questions as the research progressed, and clarified the wording on a few questions, for example on the question on sex with adults, which some respondents appeared to interpret to mean children having sex with adults, rather than adults having sex with adults. Other than that, overall the questions and wording remained broadly the same. The version provided here is therefore representative of what most respondents completed.

Appendix A

Minor-Attracted Adults (MAA) Daily Lives Project logo, July 2006

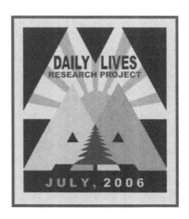

The MAA Daily Lives logo designed by a member of the paedophile community and used to advertise the project. This logo was emailed to me on 15 May 2006 and subsequently was used by the 'participant coordinators' group' and by myself on the website and materials related to the project. It was originally designed to be used for the focus-group research scheduled for July 2006. The design of the logo discreetly incorporates pink and blue triangles as elements of iconography recognisable by members of the online paedophile community.

Appendix B

Information Sheet Minor-Attracted Adults Project – Research into Everyday Experiences and Views of Self-Defined Minor-Attracted Adults, February 2007

Please read and keep for future reference.

This project is being undertaken by Dr Sarah Goode, a sociologist at the University of Winchester, Hampshire, S022 4NR, UK. Sarah is the Director of the Research and Policy Centre for the Study of Faith and Well-being in Communities at the University of Winchester and can be contacted at Sarah.Goode@winchester.ac.uk or direct line 01962 827283. Information on the Research and Policy Centre can be found at www.winchester.ac.uk/faithandwellbeing.

The purpose of this project is to find out more about the experiences and views of people who are sexually attracted to minors. Data from this research will be used to inform social policy and to contribute to theory in this area. I am recruiting volunteer respondents for this research. I will be very happy to hear from you if:

1. you are aged twenty-one years or over;
2. you self-define as being sexually attracted to individuals below the age of sixteen years;
3. you wish to participate and you have read this information sheet.

Information is gathered by way of email correspondence, responses to circulated questions (which will be generated during the course of the project as interesting issues emerge), telephone discussion or face-to-face meetings in the UK. Please be aware that any correspondence which you enter into with Dr Goode may be used as research data. *All information will be treated as anonymous and confidential.* The only exceptions to this will be:

1. if the information, including any actual or chosen name, is *already in the public domain* (for example, if I use quotations from websites where the author is named on that website);
2. if you explicitly tell me in writing that you agree to your 'name' (whether actual or your chosen pseudonym) being used in the research;
3. if you disclose details of *previously unreported* criminal activity and I am able to identify you. In this case I have a duty to report you to the

authorities and my research material may be subpoenaed by a court of law. *At no time during the research process will I ask you any questions which might incriminate you and I strongly advise you not to reveal any identifying information to me unless you explicitly wish to.*

Any information given by you will be securely saved on a password-protected computer for the duration of the project and then destroyed. Material may be transcribed, and all printed transcripts will be kept securely and destroyed at the conclusion of the project. Data from this project will be published by way of academic journals and other publications and will be used to develop a deeper understanding of the experiences and views of minor-attracted adults. If you have any questions on the research, please do contact me and I will be happy to provide further details.

Appendix C
Main version of questionnaire, July 2007

Minor-Attracted Adults (MAA) Research Questions, July 2007

These questions form part of the research being conducted by a medical sociologist at a reputable university in Britain. Before responding to these questions, please read the Information Sheet which you should have received with this form. (If you do not have a copy, please contact the participant coordinator, who will be happy to provide one.) Only answer these questions if you give consent for answers to be published anonymously for research purposes.

Please answer all questions if you can but if you prefer to write 'no comment' or leave out any questions, that is fine. The research team would rather receive a half-completed questionnaire from you than miss learning about your experiences altogether. Write as much or as little information as you like. Please return this form to the person who emailed it to you. Many thanks for your assistance!

Please note: Some questions are being used to compare with previous research by Dr Glenn Wilson and Dr David Cox (see, for example, http://web. archive.org/web/20040407042107/home.wanadoo.nl/host/wilson_83/1_intro. htm for details).

Terminology used in this research: 'boys', 'girls', 'children', 'minors' and 'young people' means 'aged under sixteen years'; 'MAA' means 'adult (or adults) aged over twenty-one years who are sexually attracted to children'

Section I

1.1 Please give your age.

1.2   Please give your gender.

1.3   What is your nationality? What is your ethnicity?

1.4   Is English your first language? Yes/No

1.5   Are you sexually attracted to
    (a) boys;
    (b) girls;
    (c) both boys and girls?

1.6   At what age (to nearest year) are they most attractive to you?

1.7   What is the range of ages that you find attractive?
    From age ___
    to age ___

1.8   What is it about this age group that most attracts you?

1.9   How do you view the idea of sex with adults?

1.10 Describe the earliest sexual experience you can remember.

1.11 Do you have fantasies concerning relationships with children? If so, how often? What happens in these fantasies? When you have these fantasies, how do you respond? What do you do?

Section II

2.1 How do your family and friends feel about your sexual attraction to children?

2.2 Where do you generally turn for support, if you want to confide in someone about your experiences?

2.3 What books, films, people, websites and so on have been important to you in shaping your view of yourself as someone sexually attracted to children? (Please list the key ones.)
Books:

Films:

People:

Websites:

Other:

2.4 *Thinking about websites in particular, please provide the following information (adding more rows if necessary):*

Name of website	*How often do you usually visit this site?*	*How often do you usually contribute?*	*What sort of contributions do you make (e.g. articles, comments)?*	*Rate (1 = low, 10 = high) how important this site has been to you*

2.5 *In your experience, is there an active 'paedophile community' (a community of people sexually attracted to children)? Yes/No*

2.6 *Is this community Internet-based? How do people find each other? How do they stay in touch with each other?*

2.7 *If you feel there is such a community, is it an important part of your life personally?*

2.8. Would you describe yourself as a political activist in relation to your sexual identity?

Section III

3.1   If you live in a country where Criminal Records Bureau (CRB) checks are carried out, have you yourself been CRB checked? Yes/No. Have you ever avoided applying for a job because it might involve a CRB check? Yes/No.

3.2   Does your voluntary or paid work regularly bring you into contact with children (for example, in voluntary work, teaching music, swimming instructor, coach, Scout leader)? Yes/No.

3.3   Have you ever avoided particular work or other situations with children, to reduce temptation? Yes/No.

3.4   Have you, as part of your work, ever received specific training in child protection? Yes/No.

3.5   Have you yourself ever been involved in delivering child protection training in a work context? Yes/No.

3.6   Are you in any specific positions of responsibility in relation to children outside your immediate family? (For example, as a youth worker, teacher, police officer, social worker, minister and so on?) Yes/No.
Please indicate what kind of job you do.

3.7   Do you have any criminal convictions or police cautions relating to your sexual attraction to children? Yes/No.
If you do, what impact has this had on your life?

3.8 Have you ever been offered or received professional advice or treatment in relation to your sexual attraction to children? Yes/No.
Have you been offered professional advice or treatment in relation to your sexual attraction to children but did not receive it? Yes/No.

3.9 If you received treatment, from what kind of person or institution? What were the circumstances (voluntary or compulsory)? What were your views on this?

3.10 Would you describe yourself as 'non-contact'? Yes/No

3.11 In society generally, there is a lot of concern over child pornography. What do you personally feel is appropriate regarding visual imagery of children?

3.12 What would you like to do with children if legal restrictions were entirely removed?

3.13 Have you ever gone (or considered going) to any other countries where the situation is different – for example, where the laws are different or the age of consent is lower?

(a) Yes, I have gone on holiday.
(b) Yes, I have lived abroad or emigrated.
(c) No, but I may go in future.
(d) No, but I may emigrate in the future.
(e) No, this is not something I have done or am considering.
(f) Other...

Section IV

4.1 What sort of activities do you enjoy with children? Where do you generally meet and get to know children? In an average month, how many children usually visit your home?

4.2   What are the good things children get from relationships with adults? What are the good things adults get from relationships with children?

4.3   Are you a parent (including a step, foster or adoptive parent)? Yes/No.

4.4   Have you found yourself sexually attracted to the children in your own family? How do you feel about this?

4.5   If another adult was sexually attracted to a child in your family, how would you respond to this situation?

Section V

5.1   Did you have a religious upbringing? Yes/Yes, somewhat/No.

5.2   Are you now a member of a religious denomination? Yes/No. If so, which denomination?

5.3   Is your faith important in your life? Yes, very much/Yes, somewhat/Yes, but not much/No.

5.4   Is religion an aspect in your work, for example do you work as a minister, priest, cleric, missionary, or other employee or volunteer in a religious organisation?

5.5   Does anyone within your religious setting know about your sexual identity? What are your experiences in this situation?

Section VI

6.1   What are the key messages you would like your local community to know about people who are sexually attracted to children?

6.2 How do you think people who are sexually attracted to children should respond to public concern about child abuse and child protection issues?

6.3 If someone is sexually attracted to children and is worried that their actions may hurt a child, what do you think they should do?

6.4 Are there ways in which people who are sexually attracted to children can support one another, as a community, not to break the law or to keep children safe from harm? Do you have examples of this happening? Is this something you would like to see more of?

6.5 If you had one piece of advice to give to someone who was wondering about their sexual attraction to children, what would it be?

6.6 Are there any other questions I should have asked you, or any other information you would like me to know?

Many thanks for taking the time and trouble to answer all these questions! Your responses are much appreciated. It is possible that I might wish to ask you more questions about particular topics. If you would like to be involved further in this research, please provide me with a way to contact you (for example, a username or nick on a forum, a non-traceable email address such as hushmail, alicemail and so on) so that I can get in touch with you without breaking confidentiality.

Yes, you can contact me for further information. This is how:

References

Ainsworth, M. and Bowlby, J. (1965) *Child Care and the Growth of Love*. London: Penguin.

American Psychiatric Association (2000) *Diagnostic and Statistical Manual for Mental Disorders DSM-IV-TR*, 4th edn, revised. Arlington, VA: APA.

——(2008) 'Adjustment of Wording of the Clinical Significance Criterion for the Paraphilias'. Online. Available HTTP: http://www.psych.org/MainMenu/Research/ DSMIV/DSMIVTR/DSMIVvsDSMIVTR/SummaryofPracticeRelevantCh- angestotheDSMIVTR/Paraphilias.aspx (accessed 1 December 2008).

American Psychological Association (2001) 'Understanding Child Sexual Abuse: Education, Prevention, and Recovery: What is Child Sexual Abuse?' Online. Available HTTP: http://www.apa.org/releases/sexabuse/ (accessed 4 December 2008).

Anderson, B. (2006) *Imagined Communities*. London and New York: Verso.

Anime News Network (2005) 'Lolicon Backlash in Japan'. Posted 13 January 2005. Online. Available HTTP: http://www.animenewsnetwork.com/news/2005-01-13/loli- con-backlash-in-japan) (accessed 9 January 2009).

Armstrong, L. (1996) *Rocking the Cradle of Sexual Politics: What Happened When Women Said Incest*. London: Women's Press.

Bagshaw, G. (2002) 'Traditional Marriage Practices Among the Burrara People of North-Central Arnhem Land', unpublished report for North Australian Aboriginal Legal Aid. Quoted in R. Wild and P. Anderson (2007) *Ampe Akelyernemane Meke Mekarle: 'Little Children are Sacred': Report of the Northern Territory Board of Inquiry into the Protection of Aboriginal Children from Sexual Abuse*. Darwin, Northern Territory: Northern Territory Government, p. 69.

Bateson, G. (1972) *Steps to an Ecology of the Mind*. New York: Ballantine.

Bayer, R. (1981) *Homosexuality and American Psychiatry: The Politics of Diagnosis*. New York: Basic Books.

Bayer, R. and Spitzer, R. (1982) 'Edited Correspondence on the Status of Homo- sexuality in *DSM-III*', *Journal of the History of the Behavioral Sciences*, 18 (1): 32–52.

Beck, U. (1992) *Risk Society: Towards a New Modernity*. London, Thousand Oaks, CA and New Delhi: Sage.

Becker-Blease, K., Friend, D. and Freyd, J. (2006) 'Child Sex Abuse Perpetrators Among Male University Students', poster presented at the 22nd Annual Meeting of the International Society for Traumatic Stress Studies, Hollywood, California, 4–7 November 2006. Abstract available online. Available HTTP: http://hdl.handle.net/ 1794/4318, poster available at http://dynamic.uoregon.edu/~jjf/istss06issd06/ bbffISTSS06.pdf (accessed 3 March 2008).

Beier, K. (2004) *Prevention of Child Molestation in the Dunkelfeld: Media Release.* Published 1 October 2004. Online. Available HTTP: http://www.charite.de/ch/swsm/doc-pdf/prevention-project.pdf (accessed 9 January 2009).

Bell, J. (2003), 'I Cannot Admit What I Am to Myself', *Guardian,* G2, 23 January, pp 2–3 and 8.

Bindel, J. (2001) 'Gay Men Need to Talk Straight About Paedophilia', *Guardian,* 3 March. Online. Available HTTP: http://www.guardian.co.uk/Archive/Article/0,4273, 4145251,00.html (accessed 11 January 2009).

Bowlby, J. (1988) *A Secure Base: Parent-Child Attachment and Healthy Human Development.* New York: Basic Books.

Bridcut, J. (2006) *Britten's Children.* London: Faber and Faber.

Briere, J. and Runtz, M. (1989) 'University Males' Sexual Interest in Children: Predicting Potential Indices of "Pedophilia" in a Non-Forensic Sample', *Child Abuse and Neglect,* 13: 65–75.

British Sociological Association (2002) 'Statement of Ethical Practice'. Online. Available HTTP: http://www.britsoc.co.uk/user_doc/Statement%200f%20Ethical%20Practice. doc (accessed 1 February 2006).

Brongersma, E. (1986) *Loving Boys,* 2 vols. Elmhurst, NY: Global Academic Publishers.

Bushie, B. (n.d.) *Community Holistic Circle Healing: Hollow Water, Manitoba.* Online. Available HTTP: http://www.iirp.org/library/vt/vt_bushie.html (accessed 12 December 2008).

Cawson, P., Wattam, S. and Kelly, G. (2000) *Child Maltreatment in the United Kingdom: A Study of the Prevalence of Child Abuse and Neglect,* London: NSPCC.

Census (2001) *Census 2001: Population of England and Wales.* Online. Available HTTP: http://www.statistics.gov.uk/census2001/profiles/commentaries/people.asp (accessed 12 January 2009).

Clark, I. (2008) The Free Network Project. Online. Available HTTP: http://freenetproject. org/philosophy.html and http://freenetproject.org/whatis.html (accessed 15 February 2008).

Coomber, R. (2002) 'Signing Your Life Away? Why Research Ethics Committees (REC) Shouldn't Always Require Written Confirmation that Participants in Research Have Been Informed of the Aims of a Study and Their Rights – The Case of Criminal Populations', *Sociological Research Online* 7 (1). Online. Available HTTP: http://www.socresonline.org.uk/7/1/coomber.html (accessed 1 July 2006).

Corrupted-Justice (2005) 'PJ Supporting Hacker Under Arrest and Indictment!' Posted 23 April. Online. Available HTTP: http://www.corrupted-justice.com/article6.html (accessed 9 January 2009).

Cossins, A. (1999) 'A Reply to the NSW Royal Commission Inquiry into Paedophilia: Victim Report Studies and Child Sex Offender Profiles: A Bad Match?'. *The Australian and New Zealand Journal of Criminology* 32 (1): 42–60.

——(2000) *Masculinities, Sexualities and Child Sexual Abuse.* The Hague: Kluwer Law International.

Cox, P., Kershaw, S., and Trotter, J. (eds.) (2000) *Child Sexual Assault: Feminist Perspectives.* Basingstoke: Palgrave.

Critcher, C. (2003) *Moral Panics and the Media.* Buckingham and Philadelphia, PA: Open University Press.

Crow, G., Wiles, R., Heath, S. and Charles, V. (2006) 'Research Ethics and Data Quality, the Implications of Informed Consent', *International Journal of Social Research Methodology* 9 (2): 83–95.

Dean, C. (2004) *The Fragility of Empathy After the Holocaust.* Ithaca, NY and London: Cornell University Press.

Department of Health (2005) *The National Service Framework For Mental Health: Five Years On.* Cited on the website of the Mental Health Foundation, mental-health.org.uk (accessed 21 January 2009).

Donath, J. S. (1999) 'Identity and Deception in the Virtual Community', in M. A. Smith and P. Kollock (eds) *Communities in Cyberspace.* London and New York: Routledge, pp. 29–59.

Driver, E. and Droisen, A. (eds.) (1989) *Child Sexual Abuse: Feminist Perspectives.* Basingstoke: Macmillan.

Economic and Social Research Council (2005) *Research Ethics Framework.* Swindon: ESRC.

Eichenwald, K. (2006) 'On the Web, Pedophiles Extend their Reach', *New York Times,* 21 August. Online. Available HTTP: http://www.nytimes.com/2006/08/21/technology/21pedo.html (accessed 9 January 2009).

Eysenbach, G. and Till, J. (2001) 'Ethical Issues in Qualitative Research on Internet Communities', *British Medical Journal* 323: 1103–5.

Fedora, O, Reddon, J. R., Morrison, J. W., Fedora, S. K., Pascoe, H., Yeudall, L. T. (1992) 'Sadism and Other Paraphilias in Normal Controls and Aggressive and Nonaggressive Sex Offenders', *Archives of Sexual Behavior,* 21: 1–15. Cited in Green, R. (2002) 'Is Pedophilia a Mental Disorder?', *Archives of Sexual Behaviour* 31(6): 467–71.

Feierman, J. (ed.) (1990) *Pedophilia: Biosocial Dimensions.* New York, Springer-Verlag.

Finkelhor, D., Araji, S., Baron, L., Browne, A., Peters, S. and Wyatt, G. (1986) *A Sourcebook on Child Sexual Abuse.* Beverly Hills, CA: Sage.

Flanagan, R. (2004) 'I'm Tired of Being Forced into the Shadows by Society', *The Express-Times,* 22 February. Online. Available HTTP: http://www.nj.com/special-projects/expresstimes/index.ssf?/news/expresstimes/stories/molesters1_otherside.html. (This link now appears to be broken, 11 January 2009).

Franklin, B. and Parton, N. (1991) *Social Work, the Media and Public Relations.* London and New York: Routledge.

Freely, M. (2001) 'Polymorphous Sexuality in the Sixties', originally published 29 January 2001 in *The Independent,* The Monday Review, page 4. Online. Available HTTP: http://findarticles.com/p/articles/mi_qn4158/is_/ai_n9662207 (accessed 11 January 2009).

Freund, K. and Costell, R. (1970) 'The Structure of Erotic Preference in the Non-deviant Male', *Behaviour Research and Therapy* 8: 15–20. Cited in Green, R. (2002) 'Is Pedophilia a Mental Disorder?', *Archives of Sexual Behaviour* 31(6): 467–71.

Freund, K. and Watson, R. J. (1991) 'Assessment of the Sensitivity and Specificity of a Phallometric Test: An Update of Phallometric Diagnosis of Pedophilia', *Psychological Assessment* 3: 254–60. Cited in Green, R. (2002) 'Is Pedophilia a Mental Disorder?', *Archives of Sexual Behaviour* 31(6): 467–71.

Friday, N. (1992) *Women on Top.* London: Arrow.

——(2003) *Men in Love.* London: Arrow. (First published 1980.)

Gerhardt, S. (2004) *Why Love Matters: How Affection Shapes a Baby's Brain.* London and New York: Routledge.

Glaser, B. (1978) *Theoretical Sensitivity,* Mill Valley, CA: The Sociology Press.

Glaser, B. and Strauss, A. (1967) *The Discovery of Grounded Theory,* Chicago, IL: Aldine.

Giddens, A. (2002) *Runaway World: How Globalisation is Reshaping our Lives,* 2nd edn. London: Profile Books.

Gieles, F. (2002) 'Is Pedophilia a Mental Disorder? Discussion in Archives *of Sexual Behavior'.* Online. Available HTTP: http://home.wanadoo.nl/ipce/library_two/files/asb.htm (accessed 18 March 2008).

Global Ideas Bank (2008), comments online. Available HTTP: http://www.globalideasbank.org/site/bank/idea.php?ideaId=2403 (accessed 12 February 2008).

Goode, E. and Ben-Yehuda, N. (1994) *Moral Panics: The Social Construction of Deviance.* Oxford and Cambridge, MA: Blackwell.

Goode, S. (2000) 'Researching a Hard-To-Access and Vulnerable Population: Some Considerations On Researching Drug and Alcohol-Using Mothers', *Sociological Research Online,* 5 (1). Online. Available HTTP: http://www.socresonline.org.uk/5/1/goode.html (accessed 9 March 2009).

——(2007a) 'My Career Has Been Damaged', *The Times Higher Education Supplement,* 20 April, p. 7.

——(2007b) 'Drugs and Identity: Being a Junkie Mum', in P. Manning (ed.) *Drugs as Popular Culture: Drugs, Media and Identity in Contemporary Society.* Cullompton: Willan, pp. 211–26.

——(2008a) '"The Splendor of Little Girls": Social Constructions of Paedophiles and Child Sexual Abuse', in Nancy Billias and Agnes B. Curry (eds), *Framing Evil: Portraits of Terror and the Imagination.* Oxford: Inter-Disciplinary Press, pp. 179–90.

——(2008b) 'Paedophiles in Contemporary Culture', in Nancy Billias (ed.), *Territories of Evil.* Amsterdam and New York: Rodopi, pp. 201–22.

——(forthcoming) *Everyday Paedophiles: Living with Paedophiles in our Communities.*

Gray, J. (1992) *Men are from Mars, Women are from Venus.* London and New York: Thorsons.

Green, L. and Goode, S. (2008) 'The "Hollywood" Treatment of Paedophilia: Comparing Some Cinematic and Australian Press Constructions of Paedophilia Between 2003 and 2006', *Australian Journal of Communication* 35 (2): 71–85.

Green, R. (1972) 'Homosexuality as a Mental Illness', *International Journal of Psychiatry,* 10: 77–98.

——(2002) 'Is Pedophilia a Mental Disorder?', *Archives of Sexual Behavior* 31 (6): 467–71.

Hall, S. (2006) *Size Matters.* Boston, MA: Houghton Mifflin Company.

Haraway, D. (1988) 'Situated Knowledges: The Science Question in Feminism and the Privilege of Partial Perspective', *Feminist Studies* 14 (3): 575–99.

Harding, S. (1991) *Whose Science? Whose Knowledge? Thinking from Women's Lives.* Milton Keynes: Open University Press.

Henry, F. (2001) 'A Prescription for Change on Child Sexual Abuse', Presentation to National Advisory Council on Violence and Abuse, American Medical Association, Chicago, Ill., 1 November. Online. Available HTTP: http://www.stopitnow.com/fh_ama_speech.html (accessed 1 July 2005).

——(2005) 'Sexual Integrity: The Path to Prevention'. Plenary Talk at Advocacy in Action, 10th Annual Conference, New Mexico Crime Victims Reparation Commission, New Mexico Coalition of Sexual Assault Programs, Inc. Albuquerque, New Mexico. 1 April. Available by way of franceshenry@earthlink.net.

Herman, J. Lewis (1992) *Trauma and Recovery: The Aftermath of Violence.* New York: Basic Books.

——(2008) 'Conversations with History: Judith Herman', interview with Harry Kreisler, Institute of International Studies, University of California, Berkeley, Calif. Posted 77

February 2008. Online. Available HTTP: http://uk.youtube.com/watch?v=USTKmf-foQms (accessed 9 January 2009). (Quotations are from my own transcription of the interview.)

Hood, C., Rothstein, H. and Baldwin, R. (2004) *The Government of Risk: Understanding Risk Regulation Regimes.* Oxford: Oxford University Press.

Human Face of Pedophilia Blogspot (2008) *Pedophile Lindsay Ashford: The Fire That Burns Inside.* Posted 26 April 2008. Online. Available HTTP: http://human-face-of-pedophilia.blogspot.com/2008/04/fire-that-burns-inside.html (accessed 1 December 2008).

Hutchison, J. and Hutchison, R. (1990) 'Sexual Development at the Neurohormonal Level: The Role of Androgens', in J. Feierman (ed.) *Pedophilia: Biosocial Dimensions.* New York: Springer-Verlag, pp. 510–43.

Internet World Stats (2007) Statistics on English language use, November 2007. Online. Available HTTP: http://www.internetworldstats.com/stats7.htm (accessed 12 February 2008).

Itzin, C. (ed.) (2000) *Home Truths about Child Sexual Abuse: Influencing Policy and Practice: A Reader.* London and New York: Routledge.

Itzin, C. (2006) *Tackling the Health and Mental Health Effects of Domestic and Sexual Violence and Abuse.* University of Lincoln: joint Department of Health and National Institute for Mental Health in England, in partnership with the Home Office.

Jenkins, P. (2001) *Beyond Tolerance: Child Pornography on the Internet.* New York and London: New York University Press.

——(2009) 'Failure to Launch: Why Do Some Social Issues Fail to Detonate Moral Panics?', *British Journal of Criminology* 49: 35–47.

Jones, G. (1991) 'The Study of Intergenerational Intimacy in North America: Beyond Politics and Pedophilia', in T. Sandfort, E. Brongersma and A. van Naerssen (eds) (1991) *Male Intergenerational Intimacy: Historical, Socio-Psychological and Legal Perspectives,* New York: Harrington Park Press.

de Jonge, N. (2007) *Child Love TV: General Information Video.* Posted 13 May 2007. Online. Available HTTP: http://www.clogo.org/Child_Love_TV_20070513_GIV1.html (accessed 29 June 2007).

Kempe, R. and Kempe, C. H. (1978) *Child Abuse.* Cambridge, MA: Harvard University Press.

Kincaid, J. R. (1998) *Erotic Innocence: The Culture of Child Molesting.* Durham, MD and London: Duke University Press.

Kinsey, A., Pomeroy, W. and Martin, C. (1948) *Sexual Behavior in the Human Male.* Philadelphia, Pa.: W. B. Saunders. (Many reissues of the original text, the most recent being by Indiana University Press on 1 June 1998, to mark the book's fiftieth anniversary).

Kitzinger, J. (2004) *Framing Abuse: Media Influence and Public Understanding of Sexual Violence against Children.* London and Ann Arbor, MI: Pluto Press.

Kohlberg, L. (1981) *The Philosophy of Moral Development,* vol. I. New York: Harper & Row.

Krafft-Ebing, R. (1998) *Psychopathia Sexualis.* Complete English language translation. New York: Time Warner.

Leurs, K. (2005) 'Exploring Pedophilia: A Pragmatic Inventory of the Pedophilic Discourse Observed from a Digital Media Perspective'. Utrecht University, Communication and Information Studies, unpublished bachelor thesis, 8 July (personal communication).

Levine, J. (2002) *Harmful to Minors: The Perils of Protecting Children from Sex.* London and Minneapolis, MN: University of Minnesota Press.

Li, C. K., West, D. and Woodhouse, T. P. (1990) *Children's Sexual Encounters with Adults.* London: Duckworth.

Mars-Jones, A. (2006) 'Lie Back and Think of Britten'. Review in *The Guardian.* Posted 4 June 2006. Online. Available HTTP: http://observer.guardian.co.uk/review/story/0,1789768,00.html (accessed 4 June 2006).

Marshall, W. and Tanner, J. (1969) 'Variations in Pattern of Pubertal Changes in Girls', *Archives of Disease in Childhood* 44 (235): 291–303.

——(1970) 'Variations in Pattern of Pubertal Changes in Boys', *Archives of Disease in Childhood* 45 (239): 13–23.

Martinson, F. M. (1973) *Infant and Child Sexuality: A Sociological Perspective,* St Peter, Minn.: The Book Mark. Online Available HTTP: http://www.ipce.info/booksreborn/martinson/infant/InfantAndChildSexuality.html (accessed 15 September 2008).

McNicol, T. (2004) 'Does Comic Relief Hurt Kids? Is the Eroticization of Children in Japanese Anime a Serious Social Problem or Just a Form of Rebellion', *The Japan Times Online.* Posted 27 April 2004. Online. Available HTTP: http://search.japantimes.co.jp/cgi-bin/f120040427zg.html (accessed 9 January 2009).

Metcalf, C. (2008) 'The Establishment Paedophile: How a Monster Hid in High Society', *The Spectator,* Wednesday, 9 July. Online. Available HTTP: http://www.spectator.co.uk/the-magazine/features/826056/the-establishment-paedophile-how-a-monster-hid-in-high-society.thtml (accessed 14 November 2008).

Miller, A. (1987) *For Your Own Good: Roots of Violence in Child-Rearing.* London: Virago.

——(1995) *The Drama of Being a Child: The Search for the True Self,* 2nd edn. London: Virago.

——(2000) 'The Newly Recognised Shattering Effects of Child Abuse', in C. Itzin (ed.), *Home Truths about Child Sexual Abuse: Influencing Policy and Practice: A Reader.* London and New York: Routledge, pp. 163–5.

Ministry of Justice (2007) *Criminal Statistics 2006: England and Wales,* November.

Morrison, B. (1997) *As If.* London: Granta.

——(2002) *Things My Mother Never Told Me.* London: Chatto & Windus.

Moser, C. and Kleinplatz, P. (2003), '*DSM-IV-TR* and the Paraphilias: An Argument for Removal', paper presented at 19 May symposium sponsored by the American Psychiatric Association. Online. Available HTTP: http://www.ipce.info/library_3/files/moser_kleinpl.htm (accessed 18 March 2008).

Moulitsas, M. (2008) 'Dems, Ignore "Concern Trolls"', *The Hill.* Posted 1 September 2008. Online. Available HTTP: http://thehill.com/markos-moulitsas/dems-ignore-concern-trolls-2008-01-09.html (accessed 2 December 2008).

Mountaineer (2007) 'Activist for Pedophile Community Steps Down from Microphone and on to Campus', Gabriel Mendoza and Victor Castellanos, *Mount San Antonio College Mountaineer.* Posted 25 September. Online. Available HTTP: http://media.www.themountaineeronline.com/media/storage/paper886/news/2007/09/25/News/Activist.For.Pedophile.Community.Steps.Down.From.Microphone.And.On.To.Campus-3005953.shtml (accessed 1 December 2008).

Mythen, G. (2004) *Ulrich Beck: A Critical Introduction to the Risk Society.* London and Sterling, VA: Pluto Press.

Nagayama Hall, G., Hirschman, R. and Oliver, L. (1995) 'Sexual Arousal and Arousability to Pedophilic Stimuli in a Community Sample of Normal Men', *Behavior*

Therapy, 26: 681–94. Cited in Green, R. (2002) 'Is Pedophilia a Mental Disorder?', *Archives of Sexual Behaviour* 31(6): 467–71.

National Society for the Prevention of Cruelty to Children (2006) 'Sexual Abuse'. Online. Available HTTP: http://www.nspcc.org.uk/helpandadvice/whatchildabuse/sexualabuse/sexualabuse_wda36370.html (accessed 4 December 2008).

Nuffield Council on Bioethics (2008) *Genetics and Human Behaviour: The Ethical Context.* Online. Available HTTP: http://www.nuffieldbioethics.org/go/browseablepublications/geneticsandhb/report_416.html (accessed 9 January 2009).

O'Carroll, T. (1980) *Paedophilia: The Radical Case.* London: Peter Owen.

O'Donnell, I. and Milner, C. (2007), *Child Pornography: Crime, Computers and Society.* Cullompton: Willan.

O'Donohue, W., Regev, L. and Hagstrom, A. (2000) 'Problems with the *DSM-IV* Diagnosis of Pedophilia', *Sexual Abuse: A Journal of Research and Treatment*, 12 (2): 95–105.

Oseran, L. (2003) *American Psychiatric Association Statement: Diagnostic Criteria for Pedophilia.* Posted 17 June. Online. Available HTTP: http://www.ipce.info/library_3/files/apa_statement_jun03.htm (accessed 9 January 2009).

Pasick, A. (2004) 'File-Sharing Network Thrives Beneath the Radar', LIVEWIRE, CacheLogic. Posted 4 November. Online. Available HTTP: http://in.tech.yahoo.com/041103/137/2h04i.html (accessed 12 February 2008).

Plummer, K. (1995) *Telling Sexual Stories: Power, Change and Social Worlds.* London and New York: Routledge.

Quayle, E. and Taylor, M. (eds) (2005) *Viewing Child Pornography on the Internet: Understanding the Offence, Managing the Offender, Helping the Victims.* Lyme Regis: Russell House.

Quinsey, V., Steinman, C., Bergersen, S. and Holmes, T. (1975) 'Penile Circumference, Skin Conductance, and Ranking Responses of Child Molesters, and "Normals" to Sexual and Nonsexual Visual Stimuli', *Behavior Therapy* 6: 213–19. Cited in Green, R. (2002) 'Is Pedophilia a Mental Disorder?', *Archives of Sexual Behaviour* 31(6): 467–71.

Reid, E. (1999) 'Hierarchy and Power: Social Control in Cyberspace', in M. A. Smith and P. Kollock (eds) *Communities in Cyberspace.* London and New York: Routledge, pp. 107–33.

Richards, B. (2007) *Emotional Governance: Politics, Media and Terror.* Basingstoke: Palgrave Macmillan.

Riegel, D. (2005) '"Abused to Abuser": An Examination of New Non-Clinical and Non-Prison Data', *Journal of Psychology and Human Sexuality* 16 (4): 39–57. (Note: this appears to be the document to which the respondent referred. No other similar title could be located.)

——(2007) *Boyhood Sexual Experiences with Older Males: An Examination of Reactions and Effects Using an Internet Sample,* self-published (not peer-reviewed). Posted 12 November. Previously available at www.shfri.net/dlr/dlr.cgi. (Link appears to be broken as at 10 January 2009).

Rind, B., Tromovitch, P. and Bauserman, R. (1998) 'A Meta-Analytic Examination of Assumed Properties of Child Sexual Abuse Using College Samples', *Psychological Bulletin* 124 (1): 22–53. Online. Available HTTP: http://www.ipce.info/library_3/rbt/metaana.pdf#search=%22%22A%20meta-analytic%20examination%200f%20assumed%20properties%200f%20child%20sexual%20abuse%22 (accessed 1 September 2008).

Rossman, P. (1976) *Sexual Experience between Men and Boys.* London: Maurice Temple Smith.

Samaritans (2004) *Information Resource Pack.* Cited on the website of the Mental Health Foundation, mentalhealth.org.uk (accessed 21 January 2009).

Sandfort, T. (1987) *Boys on Their Contacts with Men: A Study of Sexually Expressed Friendship.* New York: Global Academic Publishers.

Shah, A. (2007) 'Global Computer Usage, Cell Phone Ownership Jump', *PC World.* Posted 7 October. Online. Available HTTP: http://pcworld.about.com/od/researchreports/Global-computer-usage-cell-ph.htm (accessed 11 January 2009).

Sikes, P. (2008) 'At the Eye of the Storm: An Academic('s) Experience of Moral Panic', *Qualitative Inquiry* 14 (2): 235–53.

Silverman, J. and Wilson, D. (2002) *Innocence Betrayed: Paedophilia, the Media and Society.* Cambridge: Polity.

Smiljanich, K. and Briere, J. (1996) 'Self-Reported Sexual Interest in Children: Sex Differences and Psychosocial Correlates in a University Sample', *Violence and Victims* 11 (1): 39–50.

Smith-Spark, L. (2004) 'What Is a "Right" Age of Consent?', BBC News online. Online. Available HTTP: http://news.bbc.co.uk/go/pr/fr/-/1/hi/uk/3699814.stm (accessed 1 September 2007).

Spender, D. (1980) *Man Made Language.* London: Routledge and Kegan Paul.

Stern, D. (2000) *The Interpersonal World of the Infant: A View from Psychoanalysis and Development Psychology.* New York: Basic Books.

Strauss, A. (1987) *Qualitative Analysis for Social Scientists.* Cambridge: Cambridge University Press.

Strauss, A. and Corbin, J. (1990) *Basics of Qualitative Research.* Newbury Park, CA: Sage.

——(1997) *Grounded Theory in Practice.* London: Sage.

'Stripey' (2007) 'Are you an anime-lolicon that could turn into a RL-pedo?', Posted 4 December, in Fun Lists. Online. Available HTTP: http://hontouni.com/taihendesu/?p=579 (accessed 15 February 2008).

'Taleyran' (2008) 'More Movies Dealing with This Problem?', post on the *Internet Movie Database* (IMDb) Message Board. Online. Available HTTP: http://www.imdb.com/title/tt0361127/board/nest/97886745 (accessed August 2008).

Taylor, A. (2004) 'Child Protection: Sex Abusers Freed Because Evidence from Children Fails to Convince Juries', *Community Care,* 25 November–1 December: 16–17.

Taylor, M. and Quayle, E. (2003) *Child Pornography: An Internet Crime.* Hove: Brunner-Routledge.

Thompson, K. (1998) *Moral Panics.* London and New York: Routledge.

Truman, C. (2003) 'Ethics and the Ruling Relations of Research Production', *Sociological Research Online* 8 (1). Online. Available HTTP: http://www.socresonline.org.uk/8/1/truman.html (accessed 4 January 2007).

Wellman, B. and Gulia, M. (1999) 'Virtual Communities as Communities: Net Surfers Don't Ride Alone', in M. A. Smith and P. Kollock (eds) *Communities in Cyberspace.* London and New York: Routledge, pp. 167–94.

Wikipedia (2008) 'Infantophilia'. Online. Available HTTP: http://en.wikipedia.org/wiki/Infantophilia (accessed 18 March 2008).

Wikisposure (2008) 'Wikipedia Campaign'. Last modified 22 June 2008. Online. Available HTTP: http://www.wikisposure.com/Wikipedia_Campaign (accessed 9 January 2009).

Wild, R. and Anderson, P. (2007) *Ampe Akelyernemane Meke Mekarle: 'Little Children are Sacred': Report of the Northern Territory Board of Inquiry into the Protection of Aboriginal Children from Sexual Abuse,* Darwin: Northern Territory Government.

Wilson, G. and Cox, D. (1983) *The Child-Lovers: A Study of Paedophiles in Society.* London: Peter Owen.

Wilson, P. (1983) *The Man They Called a Monster: Sexual Experiences Between Men and Boys.* North Ryde, NSW: Cassell.

World Health Organisation (1994) *International Classification of Diseases, Mental Disorders Section,* 10th edn. Geneva: World Health Organisation.

——(2002) 'Sexual Violence', in *World Report on Violence and Health.* Geneva: World Health Organisation, pp. 147–74.

——(2009) *Programmes and Projects: Gender, Women and Health (GWH).* Online. Available HTTP: http://www.who.int/gender/en/ (accessed 23 January 2009).

Yates, A. (1978) 'Sex Without Shame'. Online. Available HTTP: http://www.ipce.info/booksreborn/yates/sex/SexWithoutShame.html#21556 (accessed 14 September 2008).

Zanthalon Blogspot (2007) *Zanthalon-Lindsay-Ashford.* Posted 4 May 2007. Online. Available HTTP: http://zanthalon.blogspot.com/2007/05/who-is-real-lindsay-ashford.html (accessed 1 December 2008).

Index

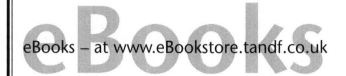

eBooks – at www.eBookstore.tandf.co.uk

A library at your fingertips!

eBooks are electronic versions of printed books. You can store them on your PC/laptop or browse them online.

They have advantages for anyone needing rapid access to a wide variety of published, copyright information.

eBooks can help your research by enabling you to bookmark chapters, annotate text and use instant searches to find specific words or phrases. Several eBook files would fit on even a small laptop or PDA.

NEW: Save money by eSubscribing: cheap, online access to any eBook for as long as you need it.

Annual subscription packages

We now offer special low-cost bulk subscriptions to packages of eBooks in certain subject areas. These are available to libraries or to individuals.

For more information please contact webmaster.ebooks@tandf.co.uk

We're continually developing the eBook concept, so keep up to date by visiting the website.

www.eBookstore.tandf.co.uk

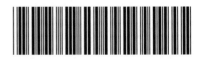